CURVES™
ON THE GO

CURVES™
ON THE GO

Gary Heavin and Carol Colman

G. P. PUTNAM'S SONS
NEW YORK

∥P

G. P. Putnam's Sons
Publishers Since 1838
a member of
Penguin Group (USA) Inc.
375 Hudson Street
New York, NY 10014

Library of Congress Cataloging-in-Publication Data

Heavin, Gary.
    Curves on the go / Gary Heavin and Carol Colman.
        p.   cm.
    ISBN 0-399-15165-6
    1. Weight loss.   2. Reducing diets—Recipes.   3. Woman—Health and hygiene.
    I. Colman, Carol.   II. Title.
    RM222.2.H34   2004   2003060515
    641.5'635—dc22

Printed in the United States of America
10   9   8   7   6   5   4   3   2   1

This book is printed on acid-free paper. ∞

BOOK DESIGN BY DEBORAH KERNER / DANCING BEARS DESIGN

This book is dedicated to my helpmate and wife, Diane.

She, like millions of other women across the land, dedicates her life to the benefit of others.

She is as beautiful on the inside as she is on the outside.

I appreciate her wisdom and indulgence as she supports me in my pursuit of truth.

ACKNOWLEDGMENTS

Much thanks to Susan Petersen Kennedy, Dick Heffernan, Liz Perl, and the entire crew at Putnam for their enthusiasm. A special thanks to Amy Hertz, a terrific editor whose creativity and vision helped make this book a reality, and to Marc Haeringer, a tireless worker who was always there to help us. Gary would like to thank his agent, Janis Vallely, for believing in this project, and Carol would like to thank her agent, Richard Curtis, for his hard work on her behalf.

A special thanks to Cathy Bergin, cofounder of Mean Mommy Publishing, Canon City, Colorado, a cook, food writer, and Curves member who created the wonderful meal plans and recipes used in this book. Cathy and her family follow the Curves meal plan in their own home, and she has made it easy for you to follow it in yours.

We are grateful to researchers Dr. Richard Krieder and Dr. Wayne Westcott, whose searches for truth are inspirational as well as helpful, and to Dr. K. Steven Whiting of the Institute of Nutritional Science, who produced the metabolic testing and many other nutritional considerations for wellness.

CONTENTS

PART THREE

EATING ON THE GO 65

CURVES™
ON THE GO

INTRODUCTION

After the publication of my book *Curves: Permanent Results Without Permanent Dieting,* I traveled around the United States, speaking about the Curves Weight-Loss and Fitness Program. I spoke at Curves centers, bookstores, and on numerous radio and television programs. I had the opportunity to meet thousands of women—many of them Curves members—who told me how Curves had helped them shed unwanted pounds, get leaner, well-toned bodies, and regain their health and self-esteem. I was prouder than ever of the important work we are doing, and the positive impact we are having on the lives of millions of women.

For the benefit of readers who are not familiar with Curves, let me explain. Curves International is a fitness franchise with over six thousand locations in the United States and ten other countries. Curves offers a unique approach to weight loss that combines nutritional guidance and an innovative workout that is not only fun, but also amazingly effective. Our goal is to make exercise easy and accessible to all women. In just a half hour, our members can do resistance training, aerobics, and stretching— the three components essential for fitness, flexibility, and *permanent* weight loss. All we ask is that you devote thirty minutes, three times a week to exercise. If you do that, and follow the easy Curves Meal Plan, you will be trim and fit and liberated from constant dieting.

I understand that for many women the notion of following a meal plan and finding time to exercise is inconceivable. One of the most memorable moments on my book tour occurred when Harriet, a woman in the audience, came up to me and said with detectable exasperation, "I'm gaining weight, and I know why I'm gaining weight. I'm gaining weight because I work too much, eat too many meals on the run, and don't have enough time to exercise. How can Curves possibly work for someone like me?"

It was a fair question, and one that I'm sure resonates with those of you who work hard—whether in the home, on the job, or both—and who are burdened with too much to do and too little personal time. Harriet's frustration confirmed something I have long believed: It's not enough to convince women they need to be fit; it's equally important to show them how to fit Curves into their over-booked lives.

I asked Harriet to write down everything she did on a typical day. Granted, she had a lot on her plate. She was the mother of a five-year-old daughter, and manager of a children's clothing shop, where she worked from nine to six. We analyzed her weekly schedule and found three thirty-minute slots that she could spend at Curves. The first was before work, right after she dropped her daughter off at school. The second was during a lunch break, when a co-worker could keep an eye on the shop. The third was after work on an evening when she had part-time child care and her husband came home early. We even found one backup time to use in case one of the other three fell through. I told her to put these "fitness appointments" in her calendar, and to regard them with the same importance she attached to her other appointments.

She grudgingly conceded that was easy enough, but that it didn't solve the eating-on-the-run problem that made her feel as if her eating was totally out of control. Too often, she said, she or her husband would resort to takeout from a fast-food restaurant. At best she would throw something together with whatever happened to be on hand.

She had a point. How *is* a woman supposed to stay on a weight-loss program when she is always on the go and has a good deal more on her mind than putting together a nutritionally correct meal? "Are you going to be there, telling me what to eat all day?" she asked.

Obviously, I can't be at her (or your) side every minute of the day, making sure that you keep your appointments with yourselves and that you choose the right foods. But *Curves on the Go,* which I designed for women like Harriet (which is, for women like you), can be right there with you.

Curves on the Go goes where you go. It makes following the Curves program easy, whether you are at work, at school, on the soccer field, in a restaurant, or on vacation. It gives you all the information you need to stick to the Curves Meal Plan, wherever your day may take you. Put it in your pocketbook, backpack, gym bag, or glove compartment.

Curves on the Go takes the guesswork out of eating out, whether you are at a fast-food or a five-star restaurant. In fact, *Curves on the Go* offers specific recommendations as to which items to order at your favorite fast-food restaurants, including the calorie and carbohydrate contents of each.

Snacking is a cinch with *Curves on the Go.* We provide a detailed list of acceptable, portable, and, by the way, delicious

Curves snacks to eat anywhere, anytime. We also provide a Dining Out Diary to help you keep track of those meals.

Curves on the Go includes a handy weekly calendar where women can "schedule" their exercise appointments, and keep track of their weight loss.

Although *Curves on the Go* is written for the thousands of women who are already familiar with the basics and benefits of the Curves program, we've included introductory information that will enable new readers to begin the program. For more in-depth information, I refer you to my book *Curves: Permanent Weight Loss Without Permanent Dieting.*

We at Curves care about the health of women and girls. Accordingly, *Curves on the Go* provides lifesaving information on women's health issues, including heart disease, stroke, and menopause.

Curves on the Go is designed to make your life easier and healthier. Take it with you wherever you go.

May God bless you with peace, joy, and abundance. See you at Curves.

—GARY HEAVIN

The Curves Weight-Loss and Fitness Plan

The Curves Weight-Loss and Fitness Plan consists of two equally important components: a unique weight-loss program, and an innovative workout that is fun, fast, and effective. In combination with the Curves Meal Plan, the right exercise will free you from dieting, once and for all. Our promise is Permanent Results Without Permanent Dieting, and we mean it!

We also recommend nutritional supplements to promote fat loss and achieve optimal health. For your convenience, we have included on page 61 a chart that describes the supplements that I recommend you take daily.

PART ONE

Fitting in Fitness

FINDING THE TIME

B ut I don't have the time to exercise!"

Not true. Anyone can find thirty minutes, three times a week. It's a matter of organization and planning.

"I'm always running somewhere with the kids. . . ."

But what about the times during the day when you're not with them? When they're at a play date, or at school or an after-school activity?

"Between work and running a home, I can't even catch my breath."

What about before work, during your lunch hour, after work, or on weekends?

"I'm always exhausted. . . . I can't work out!"

If you worked out, you wouldn't always be exhausted.

"I can't get to Curves after work. I have to run home to walk the dog!"

So that your dog can be in better shape than you? Hire a high school kid to walk your dog a few days a week!

Trust me, whatever excuse you can make for not having the time to exercise, I've heard it all before. If you visit any of the six thousand Curves centers, you will find women with busy lives just like yours—with demanding jobs, families to tend to, and homes to run—who manage to work out at least three times a week. How do they do it? Through the years, I have observed that women who do the best on the Curves program are the ones who have made exercise a part of their daily routine. They have managed their time so that they can work out on the same day, at the same time, week after week. Working out has become as natural a part of their day as going to the supermarket, dropping their kids off at school, going to the office, or even brushing their teeth. They wouldn't think of missing their exercise appointments. If a *real* emergency crops up, they make up the time.

Granted, it may be more difficult for some women to fit in fitness than for others, but it's never impossible. Even the busiest woman has "black holes," wasted time in her day when she can squeeze in a thirty-minute workout. If you absolutely can't get to Curves, you can do the Curves at Home Workout I describe in detail in *Curves: Permanent Weight-Loss Without Permanent Dieting.* Working out at home is better than not working out at all, but it is not nearly as much fun as doing it at Curves. Women with small children take note: You are typically the ones who are most resistant to making a commitment to exercise, yet you are the ones who can benefit the most from the camaraderie of working out with other women and getting out of the house for a while. Don't feel guilty about taking some time off for you. When you return home to your family, you will feel energized and refreshed and will be better able to manage the demands of home and kids.

So how do you figure out your personal best time for working out? Take the following quiz to help you determine how to fit fitness into your life.

1. If you work outside the home, can you wake up forty-five minutes earlier on some mornings to work out before work?

   Yes _____ *No* _____ *How many times per week?* _____

2. If you are a working mother, can you drop off your children at day care or school a half hour early, or have the sitter arrive early?

   Yes _____ *No* _____ *How many times per week?* _____

3. If you work outside the home, can you work out during your lunch hour? (Bring lunch with you and eat it after your workout?)

   Yes _____ *No* _____ *How many times per week?* _____

4. Can you go to Curves after work on some days?

   Yes _____ *No* _____ *How many times per week?* _____

5. Can you work out on a weekend morning?

   Yes _____ *No* _____ *How many times per week?* _____

6. If you have small children, can you hire a baby-sitter to watch them once or twice a week while you exercise? Do you have a friend who would sit for your children a few times a week while you exercise, in exchange for your sitting for her children?

   Yes _____ *No* _____ *How many times per week?* _____

7. Are there days when you can work out immediately after dropping your kids off at school?

   Yes _____ *No* _____ *How many times per week?* _____

8. Are there days when you can sandwich in a workout before picking up your kids from school or after-school activities?

   Yes _____ *No* _____ *How many times per week?* _____

9. Are there nights when your husband gets home early enough so he can stay with the kids while you work out?

   Yes _____ *No* _____ *How many times per week?* _____

10. Are there times during the week when you find yourself watching TV or chatting on the phone when you could be exercising? Be honest!

   Yes _____ *No* _____ *How many times per week?* _____

When you have completed the questionnaire, add up the number of times per week that you said you could work out. I will bet that when pressed, most of you came up with more than three possible times in your week. Now, I'm going to ask you to eliminate the times that are least convenient for you. For example, if you said that you could work out mornings before work on Tuesday, but you have a boss who frequently calls early morning meetings every other Tuesday, chances are you'll end up skipping your workout on all Tuesdays. So cross that day off and pick another day instead.

When you have narrowed it down to the three best times for your workout, fill them in on the chart below. Respect your workout appointments; don't break them unless it is for a true emergency. Try to have a backup appointment each week so that if you miss a workout session, you will be able to make it up during the same week.

KEEP YOUR APPOINTMENTS WITH YOURSELF

At the beginning of each week, set aside thirty minutes, three times a week for exercise. Write down the day and time that you will work out in My Exercise Diary below. (Turn to page 13 for extra copies.) Treat these appointments with yourself like they are real appointments—do not break them lightly. If you are forced to miss an exercise session, schedule another one immediately. (There are extra copies of My Exercise Diary on page 111.)

APPOINTMENTS WITH MYSELF:
My Exercise Diary

_____ , 200___

Sunday	Monday	Tuesday	Wednesday	Thursday	Friday	Saturday	Weekly Weight

THE THREE COMPONENTS OF FITNESS

There are three equally important components to a good workout: strength training, aerobics (cardio), and stretching. The Curves Weight-Loss and Fitness Program incorporates all three into your thirty-minute, three-day-a-week workout.

1. STRENGTH TRAINING.

Strength training is essential to preserve muscle when you are on a weight-loss diet.

Strength training means that you are working your muscles at a greater intensity than they are used to working. Working against resistance that is too light or too easy does not make muscle, and muscle is what you need to develop to shed those excess pounds and keep them off permanently. When you are on a standard weight-loss diet, you can lose as much lean muscle mass as you lose fat! The end result is, you may be thinner, but you'll also be a lot flabbier. And since you're losing muscle, you're losing the most metabolically active, calorie-burning cells in your body, making it even harder for you to keep the weight off without starving yourself. Aerobics alone will not do it. In fact, if you do a lot of aerobics, you may be chewing up even more muscle. Embarking on the Curves Fitness Program—which includes strength training—will help keep precious muscle and make new muscle. Since muscle is more compact than fat, you will look sleeker and trimmer. *Bigger muscles build a smaller body.*

2. AEROBICS.

Aerobics, or cardio (short for cardiovascular exercise), is any exercise that elevates your heart rate to your target or training level and keeps it there for at least twenty minutes. (See Target Heart Rate Chart on page 19.) Sustained aerobic activity allows your body time to access fat stores for energy. *Aerobic exercise does not build muscle.* It is an important part of an exercise regimen, but it is not the only thing you need to do.

3. STRETCHING.

After your strength training–aerobic workout, your muscles are nicely warmed up and ready for some stretching. Stretching helps to maintain more flexible, fluid joints and increases range of motion. Stretching also enhances the effectiveness of strength training, improves balance, and reduces the risk of back injury. A few minutes of stretching is all it takes to feel great.

CURVES TIP • When you stretch your muscles, ease gently into the stretch. Hold each stretch for seven seconds and gradually extend a little farther for another seven seconds. Remember not to bob, bounce, or force your stretches or you could pull a muscle.

CURVES RULES FOR WORKOUTS THAT WORK

1. PUT ENOUGH *WORK* IN YOUR WORKOUT.

There is only one way to make new muscle and protect existing muscle. You have to make your muscles work harder than they are used to working. Working at a resistance that is too light or too easy will not make or preserve muscle.

2. WORK AT YOUR TARGET HEART RATE—NOT BELOW, NOT ABOVE.

Cardio is a great way to give your heart and lungs a good workout, but don't overdo it. You should work at a pace that is challenging and not exhausting. Your target rate, which is based on your age and general physical condition, is the best guide to help you find the right level of exertion. To find your target heart rate, use the handy chart on page 19. Don't fall below your target heart rate, because you won't get a good aerobic workout; you'll be wasting your time. Don't exceed your target heart rate, because you'll wear out too soon.

3. NO MATTER HOW GOOD YOU GET, YOUR TARGET HEART RATE DOESN'T CHANGE.

Many women mistakenly believe that they should keep increasing their target heart rate as they become more fit. This is wrong and, in fact, can be dangerous. As you become more conditioned, you actually have to work *harder* to sustain your target heart rate. Your heart has become accustomed to the extra work load and does not speed up as rapidly. Therefore, trying to exceed your target heart rate could put a strain on your heart.

4. THERE'S A RIGHT WAY AND A WRONG WAY TO LOWER YOUR HEART RATE IF IT GETS TOO HIGH.

There are two ways to lower your heart rate while you are working out at Curves. One way is to simply do the strength training more slowly, and that's what a lot of people do, but it's wrong. The problem with hydraulics is that you get your resistance from the speed of movement, so if you slow down too much, you're only working at about 40 to 50 percent of your true strength, which is not strength training. *Strength training requires that you move a resistance that is 60 to 80 percent of your maximum working ability.* You have to work your muscles harder than normal to make them stronger.

There's a better way to lower your target heart rate that doesn't jeopardize the effectiveness of your workout. You *hesitate.* When your heart rate is too high, when you move to the next machine or the next exercise at home, just sit for five seconds and do nothing. Just rest. After the brief respite, you can once again move aggressively at the level that you need to overload the muscles. You've just reduced the amount of work that you're doing by 16 percent—that's what five seconds out of the thirty seconds adds up to—and that will lower your heart rate very effectively. The good part is, your heart rate goes down without sacrificing strength training. Some of you may have to hesitate as much as ten seconds before you begin to move aggressively, and that of course has reduced your work by one-third. Even that long a rest won't significantly alter your strength training. You're still moving six, seven, eight repetitions of your exercise machine at a very heavy resistance so that you're still overloading the muscle. In contrast, if you did twelve repetitions at 40 percent of your true strength, you've done a good aerobic workout, but you're missing the strength training. Remember, it's not just the amount of time you spend exercising, it's also the intensity with which you do it.

5. KEEP CHALLENGING YOURSELF.

As you become stronger, you need to work harder to maintain your muscle. Remember, if you don't work at 60 percent of your maximum ability, you will not get stronger, and you're not doing strength training; you are doing a purely aerobic workout. If you were doing eight to ten repetitions on a given machine when you first started at Curves, you should now be up to twelve to fourteen repetitions, and you should be working harder and harder. If the workout seems easy to you, it's because you're not exerting yourself enough. The machines are able to challenge anybody.

6. THREE DAYS OF STRENGTH TRAINING IS ENOUGH.

Many of our longtime members love to come to Curves and want to come every day. The problem is, when you strength train, you should take a day off in between workouts to allow your muscles time to fully recover. There's a simple solution. Do your strength training Monday, Wednesday, and Friday, and do

TARGET HEART RATE CHART
(10 Second Count)

Curves®

Find your pulse with either of the two methods. Count the number of times your heart beats during 10 seconds starting with zero. The 50% level of intensity is for special populations with conditions such as pregnancy, hypertension and obesity. Choose the target heart rate level that is appropriate for you. Always err to the side of caution. You should seek the advice of a physician before beginning any exercise program.

Carotid Pulse
To find and count the carotid pulse, place the index and middle fingers gently on the side of the neck, next to the throat. Be careful to press down lightly.

Radial Pulse
The radial pulse can be found by placing the first two fingers lightly over the radial artery of the wrist. It is directly in line with the thumb.

AGE	50%	60%	70%	80%	85%
15	17	21	24	27	29
20	17	20	23	27	28
25	16	19	23	26	28
30	16	19	22	25	27
35	15	19	22	25	26
40	15	18	21	24	26
45	15	18	20	23	25
50	14	17	20	23	24
55	14	17	19	22	23
60	13	16	19	21	23
65	13	16	18	21	22
70	13	15	18	20	21
75	12	15	17	19	21
80	12	14	16	19	20

a purely aerobic workout on the other two days. You still go through the Curves circuit, but you work at half of or less than your maximum ability. In other words, you take it easy on the machines, but you still keep your target heart rate elevated.

CURVES TIP • If you are just beginning an exercise regimen or have a health problem such as diabetes, high blood pressure, or heart disease, you should work at the lower level (50 percent). Therefore, if you are fifty years old, you would determine your training heart rate by subtracting 50 from 220, and then multiplying that number by 50 percent. You may be able to work up to 60 to 70 percent of your maximum heart rate within a few weeks as your doctor allows. Of course, check with your physician before doing these or any other exercises.

PART TWO

The Curves Meal Plan

AT A GLANCE:
THE CURVES MEAL PLAN

TWO MEAL PLANS.

Not everyone can lose weight following the same diet. That's why we offer two different meal plans. The first, the Carbohydrate Sensitive Plan, is for people who are carbohydrate-intolerant; that is, they have eaten too many carbohydrates (starchy or sugary foods) for too long. When they stop eating carbs and fill their plates with protein foods (meat, fish, eggs, and dairy products), they lose weight. Carbohydrate Sensitive people can eat all the protein they want and still shed unwanted pounds, if they limit their carbohydrate intake. (If you know you are Carbohydrate Sensitive, turn to page 28.)

The second meal plan, the Calorie Sensitive Plan, is for people who can only lose weight by limiting their intake of calories. These people actually *gain* weight on an all-you-can-eat protein diet. If you have ever been on a high-protein, low-carb diet but did not lose weight, chances are it's because you are Calorie Sensitive. (If you know you are Calorie Sensitive, turn to page 32. If you don't know which plan is best for you, take the quiz in my book *Curves: Permanent Weight Loss Without Permanent Dieting.*)

THREE PHASES.

Both versions of the Curves Meal Plan are divided into three distinct phases:

PHASE 1 is the most restrictive phase of the meal plan, but you do not stay on it for more than two weeks at a time. It jump-starts your weight-loss program by shifting your body quickly into fat-burning mode.

PHASE 2 allows for more generous amounts of food; you stay on Phase 2 until you reach your weight-loss goals, with some exceptions.

PHASE 3 is not a weight-loss diet or a maintenance program. It is a Real Life Eating Plan in which you make your own food choices. You can eat normally (and, I hope, healthfully) for most of the time, and need to diet only a few days a month to burn off excess fat. The purpose of Phase 3 is to increase your metabolism so that you do not regain the weight you worked so hard to lose.

Women who have a great deal of weight to lose (more than fifty pounds) may have to cycle through the three phases of the Curves Meal Plan more than once to achieve their weight-loss goals.

SIX MEALS.

The Curves Meal Plan provides for six smaller meals daily rather than the usual "Big Three." If you can't get used to the idea of six meals, think of it as three meals and three snacks. Why six meals? First, because eating smaller amounts throughout the day helps keep your metabolism in high gear. Second, because keeping your body fueled with the right nutrients helps to prevent food cravings and to eliminate that desperate "I don't care, I'm so hungry I could eat anything right now!" feeling that can sabotage your weight-loss efforts.

ONE IMPORTANT GOAL: A STRONGER METABOLISM.

The Curves Weight-Loss and Fitness Program gets your metabolism to work with you, not against you. In this respect, the Curves Meal Plan is different from other diets. Our goal is not just weight loss, it's *permanent results without permanent dieting*. In order to keep the unwanted weight off for good, you need to keep your metabolism working at an optimal level. This is no easy feat, because any weight-loss program is going to slow down your metabolism, making it harder to burn off fat and excess calories. Why? Within seventy-two hours of starting a diet, your body begins to produce special hormones—called starvation hormones—that enable you to survive on fewer calories. This is nature's way of protecting us from starving to death during times of famine. Starvation hormones were great for our cave-dwelling ancestors, who might have been deprived of adequate food for extended periods of time, but are not so great for twenty-first-century Americans who enjoy an abundance of food. Starvation hormones shift your metabolism into low gear and keep it there, making it harder to lose weight even though you are eating less. Once your metabolism is turned down, it is much harder to lose weight, and even harder to maintain your weight loss. It's no wonder that 95 percent of all dieters regain the weight they lose within a year!

The Curves Weight-Loss and Fitness Program is an alternative to the standard low-calorie diet that destroys your metabolism and condemns you to a life of dieting. By the time you have completed the Curves Weight-Loss and Fitness Program, *your metabolism actually increases,* allowing you to eat more food without gaining weight. What are we doing right?

- The Curves Workout helps preserve old muscle and build new muscle, which is critical for your success. Muscle is the most metabolically active tissue in the body and is constantly burning fat and calories. *The more muscle you have, the higher your metabolism.*
- On the Curves Meal Plan, you can eat ample amounts of protein to feed your muscles. You also limit carbs to prevent insulin levels from blocking access to fat stores. You'll feed your muscles while starving your fat cells!
- Phase 3 of the Curves Meal Plan is specifically designed to *retrain* your metabolism to accommodate more food without adding extra pounds. Over time, your body adjusts to eating a normal (and generous) amount of calories, and you are no longer at the mercy of a sluggish metabolism. That's why you can resume normal eating after you've reached your desired weight, and that's why you don't have to spend the rest of your life on a diet.

THE METABOLIC TUNE-UP

If you have a history of yo-yo dieting, your metabolism may be stuck in low gear, making it extremely difficult, if not impossible, for you to take off excess weight. In fact, the more you try to diet, the worse off you may be. There is a solution: the Metabolic Tune-Up. It's an easy way to fix your broken metabolism so that you can begin to lose weight again. You can go on the Metabolic Tune-Up for two to three months, or as long as it takes to reinvigorate your metabolism. (To learn whether you need a Metabolic Tune-Up, see page 39.)

CAUTION: If you have kidney or liver problems, are diabetic, or are pregnant, you should consult your doctor before going on any weight-loss program, especially one that is high in protein and low in carbohydrates.

AT A GLANCE:
THE CARBOHYDRATE
SENSITIVE PLAN

You keep track of your daily carbohydrate intake. (For the carbohydrate and calorie content of commonly eaten foods, see pages 46–54.)

Phase 1

GOALS: • RAPID WEIGHT LOSS.
• LEARN TO CONTROL YOUR WEIGHT.
• GET OFF TO A GREAT START.

HOW LONG: TWO WEEKS IF YOU HAVE MORE THAN TWENTY POUNDS TO LOSE. IF LESS, ONE WEEK.

WHAT CAN I EAT?

PROTEIN • Unlimited amounts of protein daily (including lean meats, cheeses, eggs, seafood, and poultry). You don't count calories.

CARBOHYDRATES • Do not exceed 20 grams of carbohydrates daily.

FREE FOODS • Free foods are foods that you can eat in unlimited amounts, and you do not include them in your carbohydrate count. (See page 43 for a list of Free Foods.) Free Foods include one Curves protein shake daily (see page 67).

DRINK AT LEAST EIGHT GLASSES OF WATER DAILY • When fat is burned as fuel, which is what happens on a high-protein diet, it produces by-products called ketones. Ketones build up in the body and are eventually eliminated in the form of urine, sweat, or breath. Since this may force your kidneys to work harder, you must drink at least eight glasses of water daily to flush the ketones from your body.

HOW LONG DO I STAY IN PHASE 1?

- If you have fewer than twenty pounds to lose, follow Phase 1 for only one week.
- If you have more than twenty pounds to lose, stay on Phase 1 for two weeks. At the end of two weeks, move on to Phase 2.

WHAT IF I DON'T LOSE ENOUGH?

Although most women will lose a substantial amount of weight on Phase 1 (between six to ten pounds), a small minority may not.

- If you have not lost at least three pounds the first week, and fewer than two pounds the second week, switch to the Calorie Sensitive plan (see page 32). If after another week you still haven't lost at least three pounds, go to The Metabolic Tune-Up for a metabolic adjustment (see page 39).

WHERE DO I GO FROM HERE?

Go to Phase 2.

Phase 2

GOAL: LOSE ONE TO TWO POUNDS OF FAT EACH WEEK.

HOW LONG: UNTIL YOU REACH YOUR DESIRED WEIGHT, YOU PLATEAU, OR YOU NEED A BREAK FROM THE PROGRAM.

WHAT CAN I EAT?

PROTEIN • Continue to eat an unlimited amount of protein.

CARBOHYDRATE • Increase your carbohydrate intake to between 40 and 60 grams daily.

FREE FOODS • You can still eat unlimited quantities of Free Foods and one protein shake daily.

HOW LONG DO I STAY IN PHASE 2?

Stay in Phase 2 until you reach your desired weight or you stop losing weight. You should lose one to two pounds a week. As long as you are steadily losing weight, stay in Phase 2 until you reach your desired weight.

WHAT IF I STOP LOSING WEIGHT?

If after a few weeks or even months in Phase 2, you stop losing one pound a week before you reach your goal, you need to change what you are doing.

- Switch to the Calorie Sensitive Plan (see page 32). If you don't lose at least a pound the first week, you need a Metabolic Tune-Up (see page 39). It could take up to a month or two to get your metabolism moving again in the right direction. Once you have corrected your metabolism, start on Phase 1.

- People who have twenty or more pounds to lose may have to cycle through the phases several times before they achieve their desired goal, periodically stopping for a Metabolic Tune-Up (see page 39).

PROBLEM: WHAT IF I WANT TIME OUT?

If you need some time off from your weight-loss plan, give yourself a Metabolic Tune-Up (see page 39). When you are ready to resume your weight-loss regimen, go back to Phase 1.

WHERE DO I GO FROM HERE?

Go to Phase 3 (see page 36).

KEEPING TRACK.

Count the number of carbohydrate grams that you eat for each meal and record the total on your Daily Meal Tracker chart (see page 125). You can keep track of all meals eaten outside your home in your Dining Out Diary (see page 87).

Don't forget to include beverages in your carbohydrate count. Juice, soda, and sweetened beverages contain a fair amount of sugar and a hefty amount of carbs. Your best bet—carb-free beverages such as water, plain seltzer or club soda, coffee, tea, and diet soda (if you must drink soda).

AT A GLANCE: THE CALORIE SENSITIVE PLAN

You keep track of your daily calorie and carbohydrate intake. (For the calorie and carbohydrate content of commonly eaten foods, see page 45.)

Phase 1

GOAL: • RAPID WEIGHT LOSS.
• LEARN HOW TO CONTROL YOUR WEIGHT.
• GET OFF TO A GREAT START.

HOW LONG: NO MORE THAN TWO WEEKS AT A TIME.

WHAT CAN I EAT?

CALORIES • You can eat a total of *1,200 calories daily*. That includes all meals and snacks.

CARBOHYDRATES • Do not exceed *60 grams of carbohydrate daily*.

PROTEIN • Try to consume about 40 percent of your daily calories in protein (roughly 500 calories).

FREE FOODS • Free foods are foods that you can eat in unlimited amounts, and you do not include them in your carbohydrate or calorie count (see page 43 for a list of Free Foods). Free Foods include one Curves protein shake daily (see page 67).

HOW LONG DO I STAY IN PHASE 1?

- If you have less than twenty pounds to lose, follow Phase 1 for only one week.
- If you have more than twenty pounds to lose, stay on Phase 1 for two weeks.
- At the end of two weeks, move on to Phase 2.

PROBLEM: WHAT IF I DON'T LOSE ENOUGH?

Although most women will lose a substantial amount of weight on Phase 1 (between six to ten pounds), a small minority may not.

- If you have not lost at least three pounds in the first week, or two pounds in the second week, your metabolism is stuck in low gear. You need to turn it up before you can lose weight. The solution? The Metabolic Tune-Up (see page 39) in which you will eat more food to get your metabolism moving again. (It could also be your normal monthly weight fluctuation due to water retention, so called "period pounds." If it's that time of the month, wait a few days to see if you start losing again before you go on the Metabolic Tune-Up.)

KEEPING TRACK.

Count the number of calories and carbohydrate grams for each meal and record the total on your Daily Meal Tracker chart on page 125. You can keep track of all meals eaten outside your home in your Dining Out Diary on page 87.

Don't forget to include beverages in your calorie count, if they contain calories. (Water, plain seltzer or club soda, coffee, tea, and diet soda do not, and are your best choices.)

WHERE DO I GO FROM HERE?

Go to Phase 2.

SPECIAL ADVICE FOR PHASE 1.

Phase 1 is the most restrictive part of your meal plan, but the payoff can be great. Most women lose five to seven pounds during this phase. If you eat many meals outside your home, you will have to plan ahead to make sure that you always have access to the right food. During the one to two weeks that you are in Phase 1, try to eat as many meals as you can at home, or at least "brown bag" it as much as possible. If you have to eat out (or really want someone to serve *you* a meal for a change), be sure to patronize restaurants that offer salads, vegetables, and lean protein. Order your food cooked clean, grilled, broiled, or steamed without butter or a lot of sauces. Call ahead to make sure there is something on the menu you can eat. (For more information, see tips on eating out on page 78.) And don't forget to keep track of your meals in your Dining Out Diary, or to tally your daily total calorie and carbohydrate intake on the handy charts on pages 46–54.

Phase 2

GOAL: **LOSE ONE OR TWO POUNDS OF FAT EACH WEEK.**

HOW LONG: **UNTIL YOU REACH YOUR DESIRED WEIGHT, YOU PLATEAU, OR YOU NEED A BREAK FROM THE PROGRAM.**

WHAT CAN I EAT?

CALORIES • Increase your total daily caloric intake to *1,600*, mainly in the form of protein. That means bigger servings of meat, chicken, and fish.

CARBOHYDRATES • Continue to eat up to *60 grams* of carbohydrates daily.

FREE FOODS • Unlimited amounts of Free Foods and your one protein shake daily.

HOW LONG DO I STAY IN PHASE 2?

Expect to lose about two pounds of body fat the first few weeks, and one pound every week thereafter. As long as you are steadily losing weight, stay in Phase 2 until you reach your desired weight.

PROBLEM: WHAT IF I PLATEAU?

If after a few weeks or even months in Phase 2, you stop losing one pound a week before you reach your goal, you need to raise your metabolism.

- If you have stopped losing weight, it's a sign that you need a Metabolic Tune-Up (see page 39). After you have corrected your metabolism, go back to Phase 1 and cycle through the program again.

- People who have twenty or more pounds to lose may have to cycle through the phases several times before they achieve their desired goal, periodically stopping for a Metabolic Tune-Up (see page 39).

PROBLEM: WHAT IF I WANT TIME OUT?

If you need some time off from your weight-loss plan, give yourself a Metabolic Tune-Up (see page 39). When you are ready to resume your weight-loss regimen, go back to Phase 1.

WHERE DO I GO FROM HERE?

Go to Phase 3.

PHASE 3. RETRAINING YOUR METABOLISM

Your commitment and hard work have paid off, and you have achieved your weight-loss goals. Now the challenge is to maintain your new body without living on a low-calorie diet. Phase 3 is not a diet; it is designed to raise your metabolic rate so that you can eat a normal amount of food without gaining back the weight you lost.

Phase 3 serves another important purpose: It helps the body eliminate any residual starvation hormones that have kicked in during Phases 1 and 2. Once your body is free of starvation hormones, your metabolism can return to a healthy normal.

KEEPING TRACK.

Keep track of your weight in the Phase 3: Retraining Your Metabolism Chart on page 188.

WHAT CAN I EAT?

Eat between 2,500 and 3,000 calories daily. You can stop counting carbohydrates and calories. Please eat normally and healthfully.

HOW DOES PHASE 3 WORK?

There are three simple steps to Phase 3:

STEP 1 • Establish your low and high weight • Your current weight, that is, your post-diet weight before you start Phase 3, is your *low* weight. Weigh yourself every morning before breakfast. Start eating normally. I'm warning you ahead of time that you are going to gain a little bit of weight, and it is part of the plan. So go ahead and eat and don't get freaked out when you step on the scale again. Within a day or two, you will notice a weight gain of about three to five pounds. The added weight is mostly water and between one-half to one pound of fat. This is your *high* weight. Keep track of your weight daily in the chart below. Your goal is to stay within your low and high weight, and not gain any more weight than you can lose in about seventy-two hours of dieting.

Please note that some of you may have monthly weight fluctuations due to your menstrual periods. Women who are prone to bloating may gain an additional three pounds a few days before the start of their menstrual cycles. If you know that you are prone to gain a few pounds every month before your period, simply subtract the extra monthly weight gain from your true high weight so you don't go back to Phase 1 needlessly. In other words, those extra "period pounds" don't count.

STEP 2 • **Don't exceed your high weight** • As soon as you hit your high weight, go back to Phase 1 to burn off the fat. In Phase 1, you will quickly lose the water and fat, probably within a day or two. When you are back to your low weight, resume normal eating. *Do not stay in Phase 1 for more than seventy-two hours or you will restimulate the production of starvation hormones, which defeats the purpose of Phase 3.*

STEP 3 • **Keep going** • Weigh yourself daily. Whenever you reach your high weight, go back to Phase 1 to burn off the fat. Do not stay in Phase 1 for more than three days—as soon as you reach your low weight, start eating normally. Over a thirty-day period, you will initially notice that you are dieting six to eight days of the month, and eating normally the other twenty. As your metabolism becomes accustomed to more food, it will take longer and longer to gain those extra pounds back. Within two to three months, most women are able to eat normally for weeks at a time, and must go back to Phase 1 for only one or two days a month to maintain their weight. If your metabolism is a bit slower, it may take longer. If you party for a week and continually exceed 2,500 to 3,000 calories daily, you will find that you have to go back to Phase 1 more often to burn off the extra pounds. When you resume eating normally, you will soon be back on schedule.

The Metabolic Tune-Up

GOAL: RAISE YOUR METABOLISM SO YOU CAN
LOSE WEIGHT SUCCESSFULLY.

HOW LONG: FROM ONE TO THREE MONTHS, OR UNTIL
YOU CAN START EATING AGAIN NORMALLY
AND NOT GAIN WEIGHT.

HOW LONG DO I STAY IN PHASE 3?

Indefinitely. It is a healthy way to eat and to maintain a nor-mal weight. Enjoy the luxury of being able to eat what you want and still look and feel great. Be amazed at the low level of diet-ing it takes to maintain your success. You've earned it!

DO I NEED A METABOLIC TUNE-UP?

The answer is yes if:

- Your metabolism is in the dumps due to years of low-calorie dieting, and you are not losing weight in Phase 1.
- You've reached those frustrating plateaus in Phase 2.
- You need "time off" from your weight-loss plan.

Although the Metabolic Tune-Up is similar to Phase 3, there is one important difference. Phase 3 is designed to help you maintain your desired weight. The Metabolic Tune-Up is designed to repair years of damage inflicted on your metabolism by dieting.

HOW DOES THE METABOLIC TUNE-UP WORK?

The only way to increase your metabolism is to eat more food. So that's exactly what you're going to do. You will stop dieting and begin eating normally and healthfully until your metabolism has recovered.

There are three simple steps to the Metabolic Tune-Up:

STEP 1 • Establish your low and high weight • Your current weight is your *low* weight. Record it in the chart below. Weigh yourself every morning before breakfast. Start eating normally. Within a day or two, you will notice a weight gain of about three to five pounds. Don't be afraid. The added weight is mostly water and between one-half to one pound of fat. This is your *high* weight. Why do you gain back water? When you are on a diet, that is, when you begin to access stored energy, your body dehydrates. Some of the weight you lose is water. When you start to eat normally again, you rehydrate and regain some water. If you are a petite woman, you will regain only a few water pounds; if you are tall, you will regain up to five water pounds. Remember, it's just water! Keep track of your weight daily on your Metabolic Tune-Up Chart (see page 191 for a sample chart.) Your goal is to stay within your low and high weight, and not gain any more weight.

STEP 2 • Don't exceed your high weight • As soon as you hit your high weight, go to Phase 1 to burn off the fat. In Phase 1, you will quickly lose the water and the fat, probably within a day or two. *Do not stay in Phase 1 for more than seventy-two hours.* You will stimulate the production of starvation hormones, which will further depress your metabolism and defeat the purpose of the Metabolic Tune-Up.

STEP 3 • **Keep going** • Weigh yourself daily. Whenever you reach your high weight, go back to Phase 1 to burn off the fat. Do not stay in Phase 1 for more than three days; as soon as you reach your low weight, start eating normally. Don't assume that if you are taking off weight easily it means that it's time to go back on a weight-loss diet. If you start dieting now, you will not achieve your goal of increasing your metabolism.

HOW WILL I KNOW WHEN MY METABOLISM IS REPAIRED?

When you first start your Metabolic Tune-Up, you will notice that you are dieting six to eight days of the month, and eating normally the other twenty. As your metabolism becomes accustomed to more food, it will take longer and longer to gain those extra pounds back. You are ready to resume your weight-loss diet when you can eat normally for four weeks at a time and then lose the small amount you gain after going on Phase 1 for two to three days.

Remember, you must eat 2,500 calories a day if you want to increase your metabolism to that level. Don't be afraid to eat! Your metabolism will rise to the challenge as long as you follow the guidelines of the Metabolic Tune-Up. I know this is true from the hundreds of thousands of women who have followed my program successfully; and my observations have also been verified by scientists who study metabolism. In a groundbreaking article published in 1995 in the *New England Journal of Medicine,* researchers at Rockefeller University concluded that metabolism increases as people eat more and gain weight, and decreases as people eat less and lose weight. The culprits, of course, are those darn starvation hormones. So much for the so-called maintenance diets!

WHERE DO I GO FROM HERE?

When you have completed your Metabolic Tune-Up, if you have more than twenty pounds to lose, go back to Phase 1 for two weeks and then move on to Phase 2. If you have fewer than twenty pounds to lose, go to Phase 1 for one week and then move on to Phase 2.

KEEPING TRACK.

Keep track of your weight fluctuations in the Metabolic Tune-Up Tracking Chart. (We provide blank charts on page 191.)

FREE FOODS

Whether you are following the Carbohydrate Sensitive Plan or the Calorie Sensitive Plan, you can eat as much of these Free Foods as you want. Do not include them in your calorie or carbohydrate count.

Carry a container of your favorite Free Foods with you to munch on whenever you are hungry throughout the day.

Alfalfa sprouts

Arugula

Asparagus

Bamboo shoots

Bean sprouts (cooked or canned)

Bibb lettuce

Bok choy

Broccoli

Brussels sprouts

Cabbage, red and green

Cauliflower

Celery

Cucumber

Dill pickles
Endive
Garlic
Kale
Kohlrabi
Mushrooms
Mustard greens
Onion (not sweet)
Peppers, red, green, yellow, and orange
Radishes
Romaine lettuce
Sauerkraut
Scallions
Snow peas
Spinach
Summer squash
Watercress
Zucchini

FREE FLAVORINGS

Lemon juice
Yellow mustard

CARBOHYDRATE AND CALORIE CONTENT OF COMMON FOODS

B elow I provide a list of the calorie and carbohydrate content of commonly eaten foods. Given the variety of foods in today's supermarkets, however, it's impossible to list everything here. I recommend that you purchase one of the many food guides on the market that list the nutrient values of common foods, including the carbohydrate and calorie content. Corrine T. Netzer's *The Complete Book of Food Counts* (Dell, 2000) is an excellent choice and is worth the $7.95 investment. This guide lists many of the brand-name products that you probably use in your home. However, products can change their ingredients overnight, so you can't always count on a food guide. Fortunately, many foods come packaged with nutritional labels that help you keep track of what you are eating.

On page 55, you can record the carbohydrate and calorie content of your favorites foods on My Personal Favorites food chart.

Four ounces of meat, fish, or poultry is slightly bigger than a deck of cards or the palm of a woman's hand.	Grams of Carbohydrate	Calories
Protein		
Poultry		
Chicken breast, no skin, 4 oz.	0	124
Chicken fajita, filling, 4 oz.	0	120
Chicken hot dog, 1	3	120
Chicken sausage, 1 link	3	100
Cornish hen, no skin, ½	3	150
Turkey bacon, 2 strips	0	70
Turkey breakfast sausages, 2.5 oz. (about 3 links)	2	120
Turkey breast, deli, 4 oz. (4 slices)	4	120
Turkey breast, no skin, 4 oz. (4 slices)	0	120
Turkey hot dog, 1	4	120
Ground turkey patty, 4 oz.	0	176
Beef and Veal		
Beef tenderloin, 4 oz.	0	244
Flank steak, 3.5 oz.	0	260
Hamburger patty (93% lean), 4 oz.	0	160
Hamburger patty (96% lean), 4 oz.	0	130
Roast beef, deli, 4 oz. (4 slices)	4	120
Sirloin steak, 4 oz.	0	215
Veal loin chop, 3.5 oz.	0	284
Beef jerky, 1 oz.	4	110
Pork		
Bacon, pan broiled, 3 strips	0	110
Canadian bacon, pan broiled, 2 strips	0	87

Four ounces of meat, fish, or poultry is slightly bigger than a deck of cards or the palm of a woman's hand	Grams of Carbohydrate	Calories
Pork *(continued)*		
Ham, lean, 3 oz.	0	120
Pork chop, center cut, lean, 4 oz.	0	150
Pork loin, 4 oz.	0	150
Smoked sausage, low-fat, 4 oz.	8	220
Lamb		
Leg of lamb, 3.5 oz.	0	180
Loin chop, 3.5 oz.	0	320
Shoulder, for stew, 3.5 oz.	0	225
Game		
Buffalo burger, 4 oz.	0	120
Venison, roasted, 4 oz.	0	180
Deli		
Ham spread, 2 Tbs.	1	80
Pastrami, 2 oz. (4 thin slices)	1	90
Fish and Seafood		
Bass, 6 oz.	0	200
Cod, 6 oz.	0	140
Flounder, 6 oz.	0	160
Haddock, 6 oz.	0	150
Halibut, 6 oz.	0	240
Mackerel, 3 oz.	0	175
Orange roughy, 6 oz.	0	120
Perch, 6 oz.	0	150

Four ounces of meat, fish, or poultry is slightly bigger than a deck of cards or the palm of a woman's hand.	Grams of Carbohydrate	Calories
Fish and Seafood *(continued)*		
Pike, 6 oz.	0	150
Pollack, 6 oz.	0	200
Rainbow trout, 6 oz.	0	280
Salmon, 3 oz.	0	155
Snapper, 6 oz.	0	170
Sardines (canned, in oil), 8	0	200
Scallops, 7 oz.	0	120
Tuna, 2.8 oz. (one small can, in water)	0	100
Tuna, fresh, 6 oz.	0	185
Turbot, 6 oz.	0	160
Oysters (smoked in oil, 3-oz. can)	7	140
Eggs		
Large, 1	0	75
Tofu		
(Extra firm), 3 oz.	1	90

Dairy Products

Milk		
2% fat, 8 oz.	12	120
Half-and-half, 1 Tbs.	0	35
Skim, 8 oz.	12	84
Whipping cream, 1 Tbs.	0	52
Whole, 8 oz.	12	150

	Grams of Carbohydrate	Calories
Semi-Soft Cheese (continued)		
Pepper jack, 1 oz.	0	110
Provolone, 1 oz.	0	100
Hard Cheese		
Cheddar, 1 oz.	0	110
Colby, 1 oz.	0	110
Edam, 1 oz.	0	90
Gouda, 1 oz.	0	110
Swiss, 1 oz.	0	110
Very Hard Cheese		
Parmesan, grated, 1 Tbs.	0	28
Parmesan, shredded, ¼ cup	0	110
Romano, grated, 1 Tbs.	0	28
Other		
American, pasteurized process, 1 slice (¾ oz.)	0	80

One cup of cereal, rice, or pasta is about the size of your fist.	Grams of Carbohydrate	Calories
Grains and Starches		
Devonsher Melba Toast, 3 slices	11	50
Fajita wrapper, 1 (6" diameter)	9	45
Hamburger bun	22	130
Harvest Bakery multi-grain crackers, 2	11	70

	Grams of Carbohydrate	Calories
Yogurt		
Plain, low-fat, 8 oz.	18	150
One ounce of cheese is equal to the size of four stacked standard dice. *One slice of cheese = 1 ounce.* *Half cup cottage cheese is equal to the size of a tennis ball.* *One serving butter or cream cheese is equal to the size of your thumb from the top of the knuckle to the fingertip.*		
Soft Cheeses and Spreads		
Brie, 1 oz.	0	95
Camembert, 1 oz.	0	85
Cottage cheese (1% fat), ½ cup	5	80
Cottage cheese (2% fat), ½ cup	5	90
Cream cheese, 2 Tbs.	1	100
Cream cheese, light, 2 Tbs.	1	74
Cream cheese, vegetable, 2 Tbs.	2	90
Ricotta, ¼ cup	3	110
Butter, 1 Tbs.	0	100
Boursin cheese, 1 Tbs.	0	60
Semi-Soft Cheese		
Blue, crumbled, 1 oz. (2 Tbs.)	0	95
Brick, 1 oz.	0	110
Feta, 1 oz.	0	80
Feta, reduced-fat, crumbled, 1 Tbs.	0	15
Havarti, 1 oz.	0	120
Monterey jack, 1 oz.	0	110
Muenster, 1 oz.	0	100

One cup of cereal, rice, or pasta is about the size of your fist.	Grams of Carbohydrate	Calories
Grains and Starches (continued)		
Holland Rusk Dry toast, 1 piece	6	30
Hot dog bun	21	125
Kavi crackers, 2	15	70
Long-grain brown rice, cooked, 1 cup	45	216
Long-grain white rice, cooked, 1 cup	45	205
Oatmeal, cooked, old-fashioned, 1 cup	27	150
Pepperidge Farm light bread, 1 slice	9	45
Refried beans, traditional, ½ cup	25	120
Rye bread, deli style, 1 slice	15	150
Rye Krisp crackers, 2	11	60
Spaghetti, cooked, 1 cup	40	197
Taco shell, 1	7	50
White baked potato with skin, 1 medium	51	220
Whole wheat bread, 1 slice	12	70
Yam, cooked, ½ cup	19	79

Miscellaneous

Chocolate chips, ½ cup	52	440
Chocolate syrup, 2 Tbs.	24	100
Chocolate, unsweetened, 1 oz.	4	95
Ice cream, chocolate, ½ cup	19	160
Ice cream, French vanilla, ½ cup	15	160
Sugar, white, 1 Tbs.	12	46
Olives, 2 black colossal size	1	20
Olives, 2 green garlic, stuffed, from a jar	0	15
Popsicle, sugar-free	3	10

	Grams of Carbohydrate	Calories
Wines and Spirits		
Beer, Michelob Ultra-Low Carb	2.5	95
Brandy, 4 oz.	0	296
Wine, red, 4 oz.	0	88
Wine, white or rose, 4 oz.	6	120

Condiments

	Grams of Carbohydrate	Calories
A.1 sauce, 1 Tbs.	3	15
Barbeque sauce, 1 Tbs.	6	25
Heinz 57 sauce, 1 Tbs.	5	18
Mustard, yellow, ½ Tbs.	0	1
Salsa, 2 Tbs.	2	10
Soy sauce, 1 Tbs.	1	10
Steak sauce, Lea & Perrins, 1 Tbs.	6	25
Tabasco sauce, ¼ Tsp.	0	0
Tomato ketchup, Heinz, 1 Tbs.	6	15
Wine vinegar, 1 Tbs.	1	2
Worcestershire sauce, 1 Tsp.	1	5
Ranch salad dressing, 2 Tbs.	2	110
Blue cheese salad dressing, 2 Tbs.	1	120
Green Goddess salad dressing, 2 Tbs.	2	110
Creamy Italian salad dressing , 2 Tbs.	2	110
Hummus, 2 Tbs.	6	50

Half a cup of fruit or berries is about the size of your fist.	*Grams of Carbohydrate*	*Calories*
Fruit		
Apple, with peel, 1 small	20	80
Banana, ½ medium	13	53
Blueberries, ¼ cup	7	27
Cantaloupe, cubed, ½ cup	6	25
Cranberries, dried and sweetened, ⅓ cup	33	130
Grapefruit, ½ medium	12	46
Grapes, seedless, ½ cup	14	57
Lime juice, 1½ Tbs.	1	5
Nectarine, 1 medium	16	67
Orange, 1 medium	16	65
Orange juice, from concentrate, 8 oz.	28	110
Orange juice, fresh, 8 oz.	26	112
Orange juice, 2½ Tbs.	4	17
Peach, peeled, 1 medium	9	37
Plum, 1 medium	9	36
Raspberries, ¼ cup	4	17
Strawberries, ½ cup	6	23
Tomato, 1 medium	6	26
Watermelon, cubed, ½ cup	6	25
One ounce of seeds or nuts is equal to one moderately filled (not stuffed) handful.		
Nuts		
Almonds, roasted & salted, 1 oz.	4	180
Cashews, roasted & salted, 1 oz.	7	170

One ounce of seeds or nuts is equal to one moderately filled (not stuffed) handful.	Grams of Carbohydrate	Calories
Nuts *(continued)*		
Macadamia nuts, roasted & salted, 1 oz.	5	160
Peanuts, 1 oz.	5	160
Pecans, dry roasted, salted, 1 oz.	6	187
Pistachios, in shells, 2 oz.	7	170
Soy nuts, honey roasted, 2 Tbs.	5	58
Sunflower seed kernels, roasted & salted, 1 Tbs.	1	47
Walnuts (shelled), 1 oz.	4	190
Pumpkin seeds, 1 oz.	15	127

MY PERSONAL FAVORITES

Use this handy chart to keep track of your personal favorite foods.

	Grams of Carbohydrate	Calories

WHAT'S A PORTION?

S ince few of us walk around with food scales or rulers, you need to be able to size up your food quickly. Here are some easy ways to keep track of your portion sizes.

MEAT, FISH, POULTRY. A 4-ounce serving of meat, fish, or poultry is slightly bigger than the size of a deck of cards or the palm of a woman's hand. You will eat between 4 and 6 ounces of protein per meal.

DAIRY. A ½ cup of cottage cheese or plain yogurt is about the size of a tennis ball.

1 ounce of hard cheese is about the size of one-third of your fist or four stacked dice.

1 piece of pre-sliced cheese is about 1 ounce.

VEGETABLES. 1 cup of broccoli is about the size of your fist (from the wrist to the tip of the knuckles).

FRUIT. 1 medium-size apple or peach is about the size of a tennis ball.

½ cup of berries or cut-up fruit is half the size of your fist.

GRAINS AND CEREAL. 1 cup of pasta, rice, or cereal is about the size of your fist.

NUTS. 1 ounce of seeds or nuts equals one moderately filled (not stuffed) handful.

BUTTER. 1 teaspoon of butter or peanut butter is about the size of your thumb from the top of the knuckle to the fingertip.

AT A GLANCE:
KNOW YOUR NUTRIENTS

There are two types of nutrients—macronutrients and micronutrients. Macronutrients—protein, fat, and carbohydrates—provide us with energy. Micronutrients are vitamins and minerals required to run the body. You get them from food and supplements.

PROTEIN.
The right amount of protein is essential for the repair and maintenance of cells.

CALORIES. 4 per gram

BEST SOURCES. Lean meat, skinless poultry, most fish, eggs, low-fat or no-fat dairy products (cheese, milk, yogurt).

THE RIGHT AMOUNT. Women need a minimum of 50 to 100 grams of protein daily, and more if they are working out.

FAT.

Fat is essential for the absorption of fat-soluble vitamins A, D, E, and K. No-fat or very low-fat diets can be dangerous to your health!

CALORIES. 9 per gram

BEST SOURCES. Olive oil, omega-3 fatty acids (from fish), butter, not margarine. Avoid trans fats (hydrogenated fats) found in fried and processed foods.

THE RIGHT AMOUNT. Fat calories add up quickly, so use fat sources sparingly. But don't go on a so-called low-fat or no-fat diet. Omega-3 fatty acids and olive oil are important for mental health and protect against heart disease. They also stimulate fat burning.

CARBOHYDRATES.

Good carbohydrates are an excellent source of fiber and nutrients.

CALORIES. 4 per gram

BEST SOURCES. Carbohydrates are divided into two groups: refined and complex. Complex carbohydrates (vegetables, fruits, whole grains, beans) contain fiber, a non-nutrient food stuff that is beneficial to your health. Refined carbohydrates (processed baked goods, candy, desserts) are high in sugar and low in nutrients.

Most of the Free Foods are complex carbohydrates.

THE RIGHT AMOUNT. You can eat unlimited quantities of most vegetables. (See Free Foods on page 43.) Whole grains are good for you but also raise blood sugar levels and should be eaten in limited quantities. Processed, refined grains should be avoided.

MY DAILY MULTIVITAMIN-MINERAL SUPPLEMENT

recommend that everyone take a multivitamin daily to ensure optimal health and nutrition. Below is a list of what I feel should be in a good multivitamin at the right doses. You can buy the Curves Complete Multivitamin and Mineral Formula at Curves, or you can purchase similar products at health food stores, pharmacies, discount stores, and even supermarkets. Some brands are not as complete as others. In some cases, you may need to buy more than one product to make sure you are getting all the nutrients you need at the right doses.

Basic Multivitamin and Mineral Formula

Vitamin A	10,000 IU	*Not for pregnant women.*
Vitamin C	1,000 mg	
Vitamin D	400 IU	*If you are taking a calcium supplement with vitamin D you do not need as much D in your multivitamin.*
Vitamin E	200–400 IU	
Vitamin B$_1$ (Thiamine)	25 mg	

Vitamin B$_2$ (Riboflavin)	25 mg	
Niacin	25 mg	
Vitamin B$_6$	40 mg	
Folic Acid (Folate)	400 mcg	
Vitamin B$_{12}$	200 mcg	
Calcium	1,000–1,500 mg	
Iron	4 mg	*Women with idiopathic hemochromatosis should not take a supplement with iron.*
Magnesium	100 mg	
Zinc	15 mg	
Selenium	70–200 mcg	
Copper	2 mg	
Manganese	5 mg	
Chromium	120–200 mcg	
Potassium	100 mg	

Additional Antioxidants and Phytochemicals

If these antioxidants are not already in your multivitamin, look for an antioxidant supplement that includes the following:

Alpha lipoic acid	25 mg
Mixed citrus bioflavonoids	1,000 mg
Co Q10	30 mg
Lutein	50 mg
N-acetyl cysteine (NAC)	100 mg
Lycopene	25 mg for women/100 mg for men
Quercetin	50 mg

Essential Fatty Acids

If essential fatty acids are not included in your multivitamin, look for an essential fatty acid supplement containing omega 3, 6, and 9; 500–1,000 mg

Amino Acids

If amino acids are not included in your multivitamin, look for a supplement that includes the following: multi-predigested amino acids, 500–1,000 mg.

PART THREE

Eating on the Go

THE CURVES PROTEIN SHAKE: A GREAT ON-THE-GO SNACK OR QUICK MEAL

One of your six meals each day can be a high-protein shake, which, if prepared correctly, tastes like a terrific milk shake. The basic shake is a Free Food, so it doesn't count in your calorie or carbohydrate total. We have our own Curves shake, which is a soy-based protein shake that comes in vanilla and chocolate, but there are other brands of protein shakes on the market that you can use. *Be sure to buy a brand that contains at least 20 grams of protein and no more than 20 grams of carbohydrates.* Please try to find a brand that is low in sugar or at least does not contain sucrose, or table sugar. Some protein shakes contain artificial sweeteners. We sweeten our shake with stevia, a natural sweetener that is very low in calories, and a touch of fructose, or fruit sugar. Some protein powders contain artificial sweeteners, which in my opinion is preferable to loading up on sucrose. Beware of some premade protein shakes! Certain so-called protein shakes are no more than highly sugared, watered-down milk. You can buy flavored protein powder or plain powder at most health food stores, some supermarkets, and even at warehouse stores and discount general merchandise stores. Protein powder can be mixed with water or skim milk. For a frothy texture, mix the shake in a blender with four or five ice cubes. For variety, add 1 teaspoon of real vanilla extract (but you must add 10 calories and 1 carbohydrate gram) or 1 teaspoon pure almond extract (add 11 calories). You can also add ¼ cup of fresh berries for flavoring, but you must count the berries in your carbohydrate total for the day. Below I list some simple variations on the basic shake:

¼ to ½ teaspoon orange extract (add 11 calories and 0 carbohydrates)

⅛ to ¼ teaspoon mint extract (add 5 calories and 0 carbohydrates)

1 tablespoon brandy (add 0 carbohydrates and 32 calories)

Use 8 ounces of 1% milk for a creamier texture (add 30 calories and 0 carbohydrates)

SNACKS ON THE GO

Snacks (or mini meals) are an important part of the Curves Meal Plan. The right snack can help to keep your metabolism in high gear and prevent food cravings. The wrong snack can destroy your weight-loss efforts and just isn't worth it.

The following snacks can be bought in most grocery stores if you need to pick up something quickly. They are also easy to carry around with you to munch on during the day.

Remember to keep track of all your snacks in your Dining Out Diary on page 87. If you are on the Carbohydrate Sensitive Plan, you must keep track of your carbohydrate grams. If you are on the Calorie Sensitive Plan, you must keep track of both calories and carbohydrates.

	GRAMS OF CARBOHYDRATES	GRAMS OF CALORIES
Cheese		
Mini Babybel cheese (¾ oz.-1 serving)	0	74
String cheese (1 oz. or 1 string)	1	80
Fruit		
Apple, small	20	80
Cantaloupe, ¼ of small	12	50
Nectarine, medium	16	67
Peach, medium (peeled)	9	37
Plum, medium	9	36
Watermelon, 1-inch-thick slice, cut from a medium-size watermelon	12	50
Nuts		
Almonds (1 oz. or small handful)	4	180
Cashews (1 oz. or small handful)	7	170
Macadamia nuts (1 oz. or small handful)	5	160
Peanuts (1 oz. or small handful)	5	160
Pecans (1 oz. or small handful)	5	195
Pistachio nuts, shelled (1 oz. or small handful)	7	170
Soy nuts, honey-roasted (2 Tablespoons)	5	53
Soy nuts, barbecue (2 Tablespoons)	4	49
Protein		
Egg, hard-boiled	1	75
Beef jerky (1 oz.)	4	110
Smoked oysters in oil (3-oz. can)	7	140
Smoked sardines in tomato sauce (4-oz. can)	2	180
Other		
Black olives, colossal size (2)	1	20
Green olives, garlic-stuffed (2)	0	15
Green olives, almond stuffed (2)	1	25
Sweet		
Jell-O, sugar-free (3.25-oz. cup)	0	10
Popsicle, sugar-free	3	15

If you are able to take a little time to prepare a snack, try one of the following. These also can be made ahead and taken with you to eat later in the day.

	GRAMS OF CARBOHYDRATES	GRAMS OF CALORIES
1 stalk celery filled with 1 tablespoon Boursin cheese	0	60
1 stalk celery filled with 1 tablespoon almond butter	4	105
1 stalk celery filled with 1 tablespoon cashew butter	5	95
1 stalk celery filled with 1 tablespoon peanut butter	4	95
1 stalk celery filled with 1 tablespoon prepared hummus	3	25
1 stalk celery filled with 1 tablespoon port-wine cheese spread	2	45
1 lettuce leaf spread with 1 tablespoon deviled ham spread	0	37
1 lettuce leaf spread with 1 tablespoon Boursin cheese	0	60
1 lettuce leaf spread with 1 tablespoon vegetable cream cheese	2	50
1 lettuce leaf spread with 1 tablespoon chive & onion cream cheese	1	50

Cheese melted on crackers is a sublime snack. You need to have access to a refrigerator and a microwave to make this work well.

Crackers

Rye Krisp (2 crackers)	11	60
Melba Toast, plain (3 pieces)	11	50
Harvest Bakery Multigrain (2 crackers)	11	70
Wasa Oat and Multigrain Crispbread (1 piece)	10	50

Cheese

Brie (1 oz.)	0	95
Cheddar (1 oz.)	0	110
Gouda (1 oz.)	0	110
Havarti (1 oz.)	0	120
Monterey jack (1 oz.)	0	110
Swiss (1 oz.)	0	110

Perhaps you would enjoy a selection of free vegetables with dip. The following products are easy to buy, store, and serve as a dip.

Ranch salad dressing, 2 Tbs.	2	110
Blue cheese salad dressing, 2 Tbs.	1	120
Green Goddess salad dressing, 2 Tbs.	2	110
Creamy Italian salad dressing, 2 Tbs.	2	110
Hummus, 2 Tbs.	6	50

If you have more time, the following snack recipes are sure to please you. They can all be made ahead and kept refrigerated for a day or two.

DEVILED EGGS: Halve three hard-boiled eggs lengthwise and remove yolks. Mash yolks with 2 tablespoons mayonnaise, 1 teaspoon yellow mustard, ½ teaspoon creamy horseradish, ½ teaspoon dried parsley flakes, ⅛ teaspoon salt, and a dash of black pepper. Mix filling well, then refill eggs.
Makes three servings (two pieces each)
Calories per serving: 109
Carbs per serving: 1

HAM AND PICKLE WRAP: Pat dry two (1-ounce) slices of lean ham. Spread 1 tablespoon chive & onion cream cheese evenly over each slice of meat. Cut a dill pickle spear in half the long way and pat dry. Place 1 skinny pickle spear at the end of the meat and roll up tightly. Repeat with other slice of ham.
Makes two servings
Calories per serving: 80
Carbs per serving: 1

PASTRAMI AND ONION WRAP: Pat dry two (1-ounce) slices of pastrami. Spread 1 tablespoon garden vegetable cream cheese evenly over each slice of meat. Wash and trim 2 green onions and pat dry. Place 1 green onion at the end of the meat and roll up tightly. Repeat with the other slice of pastrami.

Makes two servings
Calories per serving: 90
Carbs per serving: 1

SPICY SHRIMP SALAD WRAP: Drain a 4.25-ounce can of tiny shrimp completely. Mix with 2 tablespoons lemon juice, 2 tablespoons mayonnaise, ½ teaspoon dried parsley flakes, ¼ teaspoon salt, and ⅛ teaspoon cayenne pepper. Divide mixture between three large lettuce leaves and roll up.

Makes three servings
Calories per serving: 73
Carbs per serving: 1

BROCCOLI SALAD WRAP: Finely chop three broccoli florets (about ¼ cup), ⅛ purple onion (about 2 tablespoons), and four pecan halves (about 1 tablespoon). Mix with 2 tablespoons sour cream. Pat dry three (1-ounce) slices roast beef. Divide mixture between meat slices and roll up.

Makes one serving
Calories per serving: 72
Carbs per serving: 1

PIZZA WRAP: Set one (¾-ounce) slice Genoa salami on a plate. Spread 1 teaspoon pizza sauce on top. Sprinkle 1 tablespoon grated Parmesan cheese on top. Microwave until hot and bubbly. Slide onto a small lettuce leaf and fold.

Makes one serving
Calories per serving: 66
Carbs per serving: 1

HELP! I'M IN A FAST-FOOD RESTAURANT

F ast-food restaurants are great for price and speed, but not so great when it comes to serving up healthy cuisine. Although many selections offered in fast-food restaurants are incompatible with the Curves Meal Plan, most fast-food chains have at least one or two meals on their menus that are acceptable. Some are even reasonably healthy! The following is a list of the best meal choices at a variety of fast-food restaurants. To make it easy for you, we have included the total carbohydrate and calorie count for each meal, *minus* the calories or carbohydrates from Free Foods. (Some of these meals may contain more carbohydrates and calories than are actually listed below, but since they are from Free Foods, they don't count on the Curves Meal Plan.)

Remember to write down what you eat in your Dining Out Diary. If you are on the Carbohydrate Sensitive Plan, be sure to write down the carbs in each meal. If you are on the Calorie Sensitive Plan, you need to keep track of both carbs and calories.

	GRAMS OF CARBOHYDRATES	GRAMS OF CALORIES
Arby's		
Grilled Chicken Caesar Salad	5	218
Turkey Club Salad	6	338
Light Italian Dressing (1 packet)	3	25
Blimpie		
Grilled Chicken Salad	4	127
Cracked Peppercorn Dressing (1 packet)	2	237
Tuna Salad	6	253
Burger King		
Scrambled Eggs and Bacon Breakfast	2	140
Regular Hamburger with ketchup and pickle (throw away top bun)	22	285
Carl's Jr.		
Charbroiled Chicken Salad	9	188
Fat-Free Italian Dressing (1 packet)	4	15
House Salad Dressing (1 packet)	3	220
Chick-Fil-A		
Char-grilled Chicken Caesar Salad	3	168
Char-grilled Chicken Garden Salad	5	168
Lite Italian Dressing (1 packet)	3	20
Diet Lemonade (9-oz. cup)	5	25
Domino's Pizza		
Thin Crust with Mushrooms, Onions and Green Peppers (¼ of medium pizza)	31	273
Thin Crust with Pepperoni (¼ of medium pizza)	31	347
Hardee's		
Chicken Strips (3)	8	120
Coleslaw (small)	8	220
Regular Roast Beef Sandwich (throw away top bun)	16	270
Jack in the Box		
Asian Chicken Salad	15	128
Low-Fat Balsamic Vinaigrette Dressing	6	40
Regular Taco	15	170

KFC

Colonel's Crispy Strips (3)	18	300
2 Original Recipe Drumsticks	8	280

Long John Silver's

Battered Fish (1 piece)	16	230
Battered Chicken (1 piece)	9	130
Small Coleslaw	10	180

McDonald's

2 Scrambled Eggs and Sausage Breakfast	1	320
Grilled Chicken Bacon Ranch Salad	8	258
Light Balsamic Vinaigrette Dressing (1 packet)	4	90
Kiddie Cone	7	45

Subway

Subway Club Salad	9	138
Fat-Free Italian Dressing	4	20
Tuna Salad	11	240
Minestrone Soup	11	70

Taco Bell

Grilled Chicken Burrito	17	410

Wendy's

Junior Bacon Cheeseburger (throw away top bun)	19	320
Grilled Chicken Sandwich (throw away top bun)	21	240
Chicken BLT Salad	7	298
Reduced-Fat Creamy Ranch Dressing	6	100

SAY NO TO LOW-CARB BARS!

• • •

People often ask me what I think of low-carb bars or so-called protein bars as snacks. Frankly, I think that they are just another source of hidden sugar. Many low-carb bars contain sugar alcohols such as malitol, sorbitol, and the sweetner glycerin. These sugars may not affect blood sugar levels as quickly as known offenders such as white flour and table sugar, but that doesn't mean that they don't eventually enter the bloodstream, or that their sugar content doesn't count. When you eat a low-carb bar with these ingredients, you are still getting a substantial amount of sugar. My advice: Steer clear of low-carb bars.

RESTAURANT
SURVIVAL TIPS

On the Curves Meal Plan, you don't have to forgo the convenience of eating out to succeed. With some planning ahead of time, you can eat out without blowing Phase 1 or Phase 2.

SELECT THE RIGHT RESTAURANT.

When you choose the restaurant, be sure there is something on the menu that you can eat. A pizzeria is a bad choice if you are on the calorie-restricted or carbohydrate-restricted program, but an Italian restaurant that offers salads and meat or fish entrees is workable. Diners are great because they typically have a wide variety of food, and serve it without a lot of fancy sauces. Asian restaurants are a great option as long as you order the steamed or lightly sauteed vegetables with fish or chicken, and avoid the deep-fried selections or food cooked in heavy sauces. Fast-food restaurants are okay as long as you order one of the entrees listed on pages 75–76, and stay within your calorie and carbohydrate guidelines. Even an all-you-can-eat buffet is fine if you're committed to sticking with the lean protein entrees with vegetables and salads. Fill your plate with your Free Foods and bypass the starches and desserts. Just make sure that the vegetables are not cooked in butter. If you find that you can't resist temptation, these are not the restaurants for you.

PLAN AHEAD.

Before you pick up the menu, have an idea of what you're going to order. Look for a lean protein option (such as grilled or broiled chicken, fish, small filet, or a turkey burger) with steamed vegetables on the side and a salad. Take advantage of your Free Foods. They will fill you up fast.

GIVE CAREFUL INSTRUCTIONS.

Start with "No bread basket, please!" if you are watching your carb and/or calorie intake, and end with "Skip the dessert tray." Let your server know that you want your food cooked "clean," without butter or sauces. Ask for any dressing or gravy to be served on the side, and use it sparingly, if at all. A tablespoon of olive oil with lemon or vinegar makes a great salad dressing and is lower in calories than most commercial dressings.

CALORIE WATCHERS: WATCH YOUR PORTION SIZES.

If you are on the Calorie Sensitive Plan, please note that many restaurants serve huge meat, poultry, and fish portions. Share the entree with someone else or cut off the right amount for your meal and ask for a doggie bag. You can use it for another meal.

DRINKS TO GO

WATER IS NUMBER 1.

When it comes to beverages, water is your best choice. Your body craves it, it has no calories, and it is essential for a healthy body. Few people drink enough water. I recommend that you carry a water bottle with you at all times, and that you drink at least eight glasses of water a day. If you are on the Carbohydrate Sensitive (higher-protein) meal plan, you *must* drink at least eight glasses of water daily because protein produces waste products that should be flushed from your system, or they could be harmful to your kidneys.

Beverages other than water can load you up with unwanted calories and carbohydrates. Soda (non-diet); sweetened, packaged iced tea; and lemonade are some of the worst offenders. Fruit juice, which is high in sugar, is not much better. If you must drink soda, drink diet soda with artificial sweetener (although I'm not a fan of anything artificial!). Unsweetened iced tea and coffee are fine as long as you don't load it up with sugar. You can use artificial sweetener if you like.

ALCOHOL.

Alcoholic beverages can be high in calories and carbohydrates. I don't recommend them for anyone in Phase 1 of the Curves Meal Plan. In Phase 2, you may enjoy an occasional drink (a glass or two of wine or beer a week), but you must include the calories and carbohydrate content of the drink in your daily total. Mixed drinks tend to be loaded with calories and carbohydrates. Stick to wine, light beer, or pure spirit. There is at least one low-carb beer on the market today that contains a mere 2.5 grams of carbs per serving, and it tastes pretty good.

Alcohol is never okay if you are pregnant or you have a drinking problem or any health problem that could be aggravated by alcohol. And, of course, drinking and driving don't mix.

EATING ON THE JOB

Here are some tips on how to make it easy to stay on the Curves Meal Plan at work:

- Carry a container of Free Foods with you at all times.
- Take a Curves protein shake (on page 67) to work with you every day. It counts as a meal.
- If you don't want to brown bag it, find a local deli or grocery with a salad bar. Fill up your plate with Free Foods, and add some lean protein to your salad, such as hard-boiled eggs or fresh turkey or ham to complete your meal.
- Save time and money. You can eat in a fast-food restaurant as long as you order one of the acceptable meals listed on pages 75–76, and stay within your calorie and carbohydrate guidelines.
- Keep individual cans of tuna (in water), salmon, or canned chicken in your desk or locker for a quick meal with your cut-up vegetables.
- If you have access to a refrigerator at work, stock it at the beginning of the week with low-fat cottage cheese, yogurt,

prepackaged salad, and other foods that will help you put together a quick meal.

- If you bring salad to work, pack the lettuce in one container
  and the wet ingredients (tomato, cucumber, etc.) in another,
  and mix them together when you are ready for your meal.
  Top your salad with some high-quality-protein leftover sliced
  steak, chicken breast, or a can of salmon or tuna. Mix in a small
  amount of oil and vinegar or your favorite low-carbohydrate
  salad dressing.

- Cook an extra portion of chicken, meat, or fish the night before to have for lunch the next day. Store it overnight in the
  same container that you will bring to work.

PART FOUR

Keeping Track

MY DINING OUT DIARY

Keep track of all meals and snacks that you eat outside your home with this handy chart. If you are on the Carbohydrate Sensitive Plan, you need to record the amount of carbohydrate grams consumed at each meal. If you are on the Calorie Sensitive Plan, you need to record the amount of both carbohydrate grams and calories consumed at each meal. For more information on each meal plan, turn to page 23.

At the end of each day, transfer the information from the chart below to your Daily Meal Tracker chart on page 125.

Below, I have provided 100 blank charts. You can download additional My Dining Out Diary pages from my website www.curvesinternational.com.

My Dining Out Diary

Date _____   CALORIES   CARBOHYDRATES
Meal _____
_____
_____
_____
                        TOTALS   _____   _____

Date _____   CALORIES   CARBOHYDRATES
Meal _____
_____
_____
_____
                        TOTALS   _____   _____

Date _____   CALORIES   CARBOHYDRATES
Meal _____
_____
_____
_____
                        TOTALS   _____   _____

Date _____   CALORIES   CARBOHYDRATES
Meal _____
_____
_____
_____
                        TOTALS   _____   _____

Date _____   CALORIES   CARBOHYDRATES
Meal _____
_____
_____
_____
                        TOTALS   _____   _____

My Dining Out Diary

Date _____

Meal _____

_____

_____

_____

CALORIES   CARBOHYDRATES

TOTALS   _____   _____

Date _____

Meal _____

_____

_____

_____

CALORIES   CARBOHYDRATES

TOTALS   _____   _____

Date _____

Meal _____

_____

_____

_____

CALORIES   CARBOHYDRATES

TOTALS   _____   _____

Date _____

Meal _____

_____

_____

_____

CALORIES   CARBOHYDRATES

TOTALS   _____   _____

Date _____

Meal _____

_____

_____

_____

CALORIES   CARBOHYDRATES

TOTALS   _____   _____

My Dining Out Diary

Date _____   CALORIES   CARBOHYDRATES
Meal _____
     _____
     _____
     _____
                          TOTALS   _____   _____

Date _____   CALORIES   CARBOHYDRATES
Meal _____
     _____
     _____
     _____
                          TOTALS   _____   _____

Date _____   CALORIES   CARBOHYDRATES
Meal _____
     _____
     _____
     _____
                          TOTALS   _____   _____

Date _____   CALORIES   CARBOHYDRATES
Meal _____
     _____
     _____
     _____
                          TOTALS   _____   _____

Date _____   CALORIES   CARBOHYDRATES
Meal _____
     _____
     _____
     _____
                          TOTALS   _____   _____

My Dining Out Diary

Date _____

Meal _____
_____
_____
_____

CALORIES   CARBOHYDRATES

TOTALS _____   _____

Date _____

Meal _____
_____
_____
_____

CALORIES   CARBOHYDRATES

TOTALS _____   _____

Date _____

Meal _____
_____
_____
_____

CALORIES   CARBOHYDRATES

TOTALS _____   _____

Date _____

Meal _____
_____
_____
_____

CALORIES   CARBOHYDRATES

TOTALS _____   _____

Date _____

Meal _____
_____
_____
_____

CALORIES   CARBOHYDRATES

TOTALS _____   _____

My Dining Out Diary

Date _____   CALORIES   CARBOHYDRATES
Meal _____
_____
_____
_____
                                TOTALS   _____   _____

Date _____   CALORIES   CARBOHYDRATES
Meal _____
_____
_____
_____
                                TOTALS   _____   _____

Date _____   CALORIES   CARBOHYDRATES
Meal _____
_____
_____
_____
                                TOTALS   _____   _____

Date _____   CALORIES   CARBOHYDRATES
Meal _____
_____
_____
_____
                                TOTALS   _____   _____

Date _____   CALORIES   CARBOHYDRATES
Meal _____
_____
_____
_____
                                TOTALS   _____   _____

My Dining Out Diary

Date _____   CALORIES   CARBOHYDRATES
Meal _____
_____
_____
_____
                              TOTALS   _____   _____

Date _____   CALORIES   CARBOHYDRATES
Meal _____
_____
_____
_____
                              TOTALS   _____   _____

Date _____   CALORIES   CARBOHYDRATES
Meal _____
_____
_____
_____
                              TOTALS   _____   _____

Date _____   CALORIES   CARBOHYDRATES
Meal _____
_____
_____
_____
                              TOTALS   _____   _____

Date _____   CALORIES   CARBOHYDRATES
Meal _____
_____
_____
_____
                              TOTALS   _____   _____

My Dining Out Diary

Date _____   CALORIES   CARBOHYDRATES
Meal _____
_____
_____
_____
                                    TOTALS   _____   _____

Date _____   CALORIES   CARBOHYDRATES
Meal _____
_____
_____
_____
                                    TOTALS   _____   _____

Date _____   CALORIES   CARBOHYDRATES
Meal _____
_____
_____
_____
                                    TOTALS   _____   _____

Date _____   CALORIES   CARBOHYDRATES
Meal _____
_____
_____
_____
                                    TOTALS   _____   _____

Date _____   CALORIES   CARBOHYDRATES
Meal _____
_____
_____
_____
                                    TOTALS   _____   _____

My Dining Out Diary

Date _____   CALORIES   CARBOHYDRATES
Meal _____
_____
_____
_____
                                    TOTALS   _____   _____

Date _____   CALORIES   CARBOHYDRATES
Meal _____
_____
_____
_____
                                    TOTALS   _____   _____

Date _____   CALORIES   CARBOHYDRATES
Meal _____
_____
_____
_____
                                    TOTALS   _____   _____

Date _____   CALORIES   CARBOHYDRATES
Meal _____
_____
_____
_____
                                    TOTALS   _____   _____

Date _____   CALORIES   CARBOHYDRATES
Meal _____
_____
_____
_____
                                    TOTALS   _____   _____

My Dining Out Diary

Date _____
Meal _____
_____
_____
_____

CALORIES   CARBOHYDRATES

TOTALS   _____   _____

Date _____
Meal _____
_____
_____
_____

CALORIES   CARBOHYDRATES

TOTALS   _____   _____

Date _____
Meal _____
_____
_____
_____

CALORIES   CARBOHYDRATES

TOTALS   _____   _____

Date _____
Meal _____
_____
_____
_____

CALORIES   CARBOHYDRATES

TOTALS   _____   _____

Date _____
Meal _____
_____
_____
_____

CALORIES   CARBOHYDRATES

TOTALS   _____   _____

My Dining Out Diary

Date _____

Meal _____

_____

_____

_____

CALORIES   CARBOHYDRATES

TOTALS _____ _____

Date _____

Meal _____

_____

_____

_____

CALORIES   CARBOHYDRATES

TOTALS _____ _____

Date _____

Meal _____

_____

_____

_____

CALORIES   CARBOHYDRATES

TOTALS _____ _____

Date _____

Meal _____

_____

_____

_____

CALORIES   CARBOHYDRATES

TOTALS _____ _____

Date _____

Meal _____

_____

_____

_____

CALORIES   CARBOHYDRATES

TOTALS _____ _____

My Dining Out Diary

Date _____   CALORIES   CARBOHYDRATES
Meal _____
_____
_____
_____
                              TOTALS   _____   _____

Date _____   CALORIES   CARBOHYDRATES
Meal _____
_____
_____
_____
                              TOTALS   _____   _____

Date _____   CALORIES   CARBOHYDRATES
Meal _____
_____
_____
_____
                              TOTALS   _____   _____

Date _____   CALORIES   CARBOHYDRATES
Meal _____
_____
_____
_____
                              TOTALS   _____   _____

Date _____   CALORIES   CARBOHYDRATES
Meal _____
_____
_____
_____
                              TOTALS   _____   _____

My Dining Out Diary

Date _____

	CALORIES	CARBOHYDRATES
Meal _____
_____
_____
_____

TOTALS _____ _____

Date _____

	CALORIES	CARBOHYDRATES
Meal _____
_____
_____
_____

TOTALS _____ _____

Date _____

	CALORIES	CARBOHYDRATES
Meal _____
_____
_____
_____

TOTALS _____ _____

Date _____

	CALORIES	CARBOHYDRATES
Meal _____
_____
_____
_____

TOTALS _____ _____

Date _____

	CALORIES	CARBOHYDRATES
Meal _____
_____
_____
_____

TOTALS _____ _____

My Dining Out Diary

Date _____
Meal _____
_____
_____
_____

CALORIES   CARBOHYDRATES

TOTALS   _____   _____

Date _____
Meal _____
_____
_____
_____

CALORIES   CARBOHYDRATES

TOTALS   _____   _____

Date _____
Meal _____
_____
_____
_____

CALORIES   CARBOHYDRATES

TOTALS   _____   _____

Date _____
Meal _____
_____
_____
_____

CALORIES   CARBOHYDRATES

TOTALS   _____   _____

Date _____
Meal _____
_____
_____
_____

CALORIES   CARBOHYDRATES

TOTALS   _____   _____

My Dining Out Diary

Date _____

Meal _____
_____
_____
_____

CALORIES   CARBOHYDRATES

TOTALS   _____   _____

Date _____

Meal _____
_____
_____
_____

CALORIES   CARBOHYDRATES

TOTALS   _____   _____

Date _____

Meal _____
_____
_____
_____

CALORIES   CARBOHYDRATES

TOTALS   _____   _____

Date _____

Meal _____
_____
_____
_____

CALORIES   CARBOHYDRATES

TOTALS   _____   _____

Date _____

Meal _____
_____
_____
_____

CALORIES   CARBOHYDRATES

TOTALS   _____   _____

My Dining Out Diary

Date _____   CALORIES   CARBOHYDRATES
Meal _____
_____
_____
_____
                                    TOTALS   _____   _____

Date _____   CALORIES   CARBOHYDRATES
Meal _____
_____
_____
_____
                                    TOTALS   _____   _____

Date _____   CALORIES   CARBOHYDRATES
Meal _____
_____
_____
_____
                                    TOTALS   _____   _____

Date _____   CALORIES   CARBOHYDRATES
Meal _____
_____
_____
_____
                                    TOTALS   _____   _____

Date _____   CALORIES   CARBOHYDRATES
Meal _____
_____
_____
_____
                                    TOTALS   _____   _____

My Dining Out Diary

Date _____

Meal _____

_____

_____

_____

CALORIES   CARBOHYDRATES

TOTALS _____   _____

Date _____

Meal _____

_____

_____

_____

CALORIES   CARBOHYDRATES

TOTALS _____   _____

Date _____

Meal _____

_____

_____

_____

CALORIES   CARBOHYDRATES

TOTALS _____   _____

Date _____

Meal _____

_____

_____

_____

CALORIES   CARBOHYDRATES

TOTALS _____   _____

Date _____

Meal _____

_____

_____

_____

CALORIES   CARBOHYDRATES

TOTALS _____   _____

My Dining Out Diary

Date _____   CALORIES   CARBOHYDRATES
Meal _____
_____
_____
_____
                                          TOTALS   _____   _____

Date _____   CALORIES   CARBOHYDRATES
Meal _____
_____
_____
_____
                                          TOTALS   _____   _____

Date _____   CALORIES   CARBOHYDRATES
Meal _____
_____
_____
_____
                                          TOTALS   _____   _____

Date _____   CALORIES   CARBOHYDRATES
Meal _____
_____
_____
_____
                                          TOTALS   _____   _____

Date _____   CALORIES   CARBOHYDRATES
Meal _____
_____
_____
_____
                                          TOTALS   _____   _____

My Dining Out Diary

Date _____   CALORIES   CARBOHYDRATES
Meal _____
_____
_____
_____
                              TOTALS   _____   _____

Date _____   CALORIES   CARBOHYDRATES
Meal _____
_____
_____
_____
                              TOTALS   _____   _____

Date _____   CALORIES   CARBOHYDRATES
Meal _____
_____
_____
_____
                              TOTALS   _____   _____

Date _____   CALORIES   CARBOHYDRATES
Meal _____
_____
_____
_____
                              TOTALS   _____   _____

Date _____   CALORIES   CARBOHYDRATES
Meal _____
_____
_____
_____
                              TOTALS   _____   _____

My Dining Out Diary

Date _____ CALORIES CARBOHYDRATES
Meal _____
     _____
     _____
     _____
                    TOTALS   _____   _____

Date _____ CALORIES CARBOHYDRATES
Meal _____
     _____
     _____
     _____
                    TOTALS   _____   _____

Date _____ CALORIES CARBOHYDRATES
Meal _____
     _____
     _____
     _____
                    TOTALS   _____   _____

Date _____ CALORIES CARBOHYDRATES
Meal _____
     _____
     _____
     _____
                    TOTALS   _____   _____

Date _____ CALORIES CARBOHYDRATES
Meal _____
     _____
     _____
     _____
                    TOTALS   _____   _____

My Dining Out Diary

Date _____   CALORIES   CARBOHYDRATES
Meal _____
     _____
     _____
     _____
                    TOTALS   _____   _____

Date _____   CALORIES   CARBOHYDRATES
Meal _____
     _____
     _____
     _____
                    TOTALS   _____   _____

Date _____   CALORIES   CARBOHYDRATES
Meal _____
     _____
     _____
     _____
                    TOTALS   _____   _____

Date _____   CALORIES   CARBOHYDRATES
Meal _____
     _____
     _____
     _____
                    TOTALS   _____   _____

Date _____   CALORIES   CARBOHYDRATES
Meal _____
     _____
     _____
     _____
                    TOTALS   _____   _____

My Dining Out Diary

Date _____   CALORIES   CARBOHYDRATES
Meal _____
_____
_____
_____
                              TOTALS   _____   _____

Date _____   CALORIES   CARBOHYDRATES
Meal _____
_____
_____
_____
                              TOTALS   _____   _____

Date _____   CALORIES   CARBOHYDRATES
Meal _____
_____
_____
_____
                              TOTALS   _____   _____

Date _____   CALORIES   CARBOHYDRATES
Meal _____
_____
_____
_____
                              TOTALS   _____   _____

Date _____   CALORIES   CARBOHYDRATES
Meal _____
_____
_____
_____
                              TOTALS   _____   _____

My Dining Out Diary

Date _____

Meal _____

_____

_____

_____

	CALORIES	CARBOHYDRATES
TOTALS	_____	_____

Date _____

Meal _____

_____

_____

_____

	CALORIES	CARBOHYDRATES
TOTALS	_____	_____

Date _____

Meal _____

_____

_____

_____

	CALORIES	CARBOHYDRATES
TOTALS	_____	_____

Date _____

Meal _____

_____

_____

_____

	CALORIES	CARBOHYDRATES
TOTALS	_____	_____

Date _____

Meal _____

_____

_____

_____

	CALORIES	CARBOHYDRATES
TOTALS	_____	_____

KEEP YOUR
APPOINTMENTS
WITH YOURSELF

A t the beginning of each week, set aside thirty minutes, three times a week for exercise. Write down the day and time that you will work out in My Exercise Diary on page 13. Treat these appointments with yourself like they are real appointments—do not break them lightly. If you are forced to miss an exercise session, schedule another one immediately.

Use this handy chart as a way of keeping track of your weight. Weigh yourself once a week, first thing in the morning before you eat. Write down your weight in the blank space below. Weigh yourself at the same time and on the same day each week.

Sunday	Monday	Tuesday	Wednesday	Thursday	Friday	

APPOINTMENTS WITH MYSELF: _____, 200__

My Exercise Diary

KEEP YOUR APPOINTMENTS WITH YOURSELF

Sunday	Monday	Tuesday	Wednesday	Thursday	Friday	Saturday	Weekly Weight

APPOINTMENTS WITH MYSELF:
My Exercise Diary

———— , 200 ————

Sunday	Monday	Tuesday	Wednesday	Thursday	Friday	Saturday	Weekly Weight

APPOINTMENTS WITH MYSELF:
My Exercise Diary

———— , 200 ————

Sunday	Monday	Tuesday	Wednesday	Thursday	Friday	Saturday	Weekly Weight

APPOINTMENTS WITH MYSELF:
My Exercise Diary

_____ , 200 ___

Sunday	Monday	Tuesday	Wednesday	Thursday	Friday	Saturday	Weekly Weight

APPOINTMENTS WITH MYSELF:

My Exercise Diary

_____ , 200 _____

Sunday	Monday	Tuesday	Wednesday	Thursday	Friday	Saturday	Weekly Weight

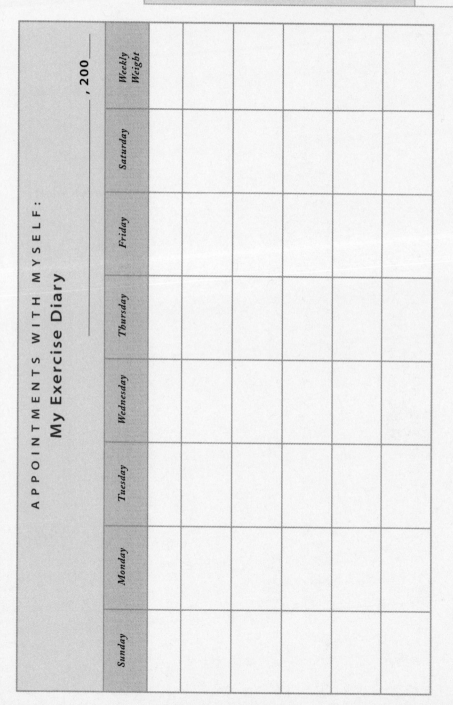

APPOINTMENTS WITH MYSELF:
My Exercise Diary

_____, 200___

Sunday	Monday	Tuesday	Wednesday	Thursday	Friday	Saturday	Weekly Weight

APPOINTMENTS WITH MYSELF:

My Exercise Diary

_____ , 200___

	Sunday	Monday	Tuesday	Wednesday	Thursday	Friday	Saturday	Weekly Weight

APPOINTMENTS WITH MYSELF:
My Exercise Diary

_____ , 200___

Sunday	Monday	Tuesday	Wednesday	Thursday	Friday	Saturday	Weekly Weight

APPOINTMENTS WITH MYSELF:

My Exercise Diary

_____, 200___

Sunday	Monday	Tuesday	Wednesday	Thursday	Friday	Saturday	Weekly Weight

APPOINTMENTS WITH MYSELF:
My Exercise Diary

_____ , 200 ____

Sunday	Monday	Tuesday	Wednesday	Thursday	Friday	Saturday	Weekly Weight

APPOINTMENTS WITH MYSELF:
My Exercise Diary

_____ , 200 ___

Sunday	Monday	Tuesday	Wednesday	Thursday	Friday	Saturday	Weekly Weight

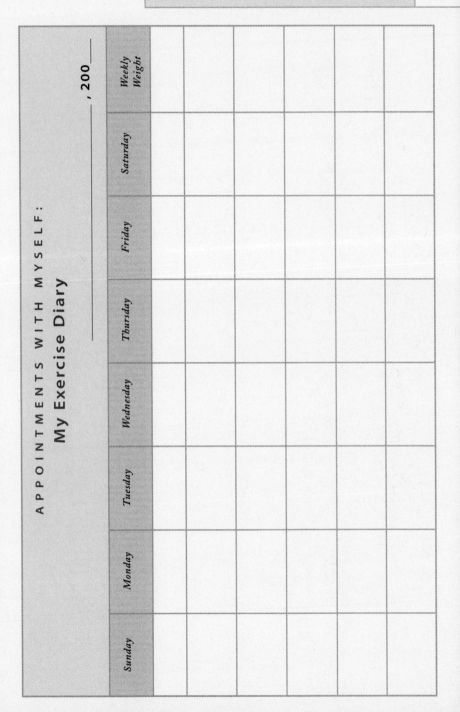

APPOINTMENTS WITH MYSELF:
My Exercise Diary

_____ , 200___

Sunday	Monday	Tuesday	Wednesday	Thursday	Friday	Saturday	Weekly Weight

APPOINTMENTS WITH MYSELF:
My Exercise Diary

_____ , 200 _____

Sunday	Monday	Tuesday	Wednesday	Thursday	Friday	Saturday	Weekly Weight

MY DAILY MEAL TRACKER

I f you are on the Carbohydrate Sensitive Plan, keep track of your daily carbohydrate intake.

PHASE 1 · Eat no more than 20 grams of carbohydrates daily.

PHASE 2 · Eat no more than 60 grams of carbohydrates daily.

I f you are on the Calorie Sensitive Plan, keep track of both your daily carbohydrate and daily calorie intake.

PHASE 1 · Eat no more than 1,200 calories and 60 grams of carbohydrates daily.

PHASE 2 · Eat no more than 1,600 calories and 60 grams of carbohydrates daily.

Free Foods do not count in your daily totals.

Date_____

Meal	Calories	Carbohydrates
1		
2		
3		
4		
5		
6		
Total:		

Date_____

Meal	Calories	Carbohydrates
1		
2		
3		
4		
5		
6		
Total:		

Date_____

Meal	Calories	Carbohydrates
1		
2		
3		
4		
5		
6		
Total:		

Date_____

Meal	Calories	Carbohydrates
1		
2		
3		
4		
5		
6		
Total:		

Date_____

Meal	Calories	Carbohydrates
1		
2		
3		
4		
5		
6		
Total:		

Date_____

Meal	Calories	Carbohydrates
1		
2		
3		
4		
5		
6		
Total:		

Date_____

Meal	Calories	Carbohydrates
1		
2		
3		
4		
5		
6		
Total:		

Date_____

Meal	Calories	Carbohydrates
1		
2		
3		
4		
5		
6		
Total:		

Date_____

Meal	Calories	Carbohydrates
1		
2		
3		
4		
5		
6		
Total:		

Date_____

Meal	Calories	Carbohydrates
1		
2		
3		
4		
5		
6		
Total:		

Date_____

Meal	Calories	Carbohydrates
1		
2		
3		
4		
5		
6		
Total:		

Date_____

Meal	Calories	Carbohydrates
1		
2		
3		
4		
5		
6		
Total:		

Date_____

Meal	Calories	Carbohydrates
1		
2		
3		
4		
5		
6		
Total:		

Date_____

Meal	Calories	Carbohydrates
1		
2		
3		
4		
5		
6		
Total:		

Date_____

Meal	Calories	Carbohydrates
1		
2		
3		
4		
5		
6		
Total:		

Date_____

Meal	Calories	Carbohydrates
1		
2		
3		
4		
5		
6		
Total:		

Date_____

Meal	Calories	Carbohydrates
1		
2		
3		
4		
5		
6		
Total:		

Date_____

Meal	Calories	Carbohydrates
1		
2		
3		
4		
5		
6		
Total:		

Date_____

Meal	Calories	Carbohydrates
1		
2		
3		
4		
5		
6		
Total:		

Date_____

Meal	Calories	Carbohydrates
1		
2		
3		
4		
5		
6		
Total:		

Date_____

Meal	Calories	Carbohydrates
1		
2		
3		
4		
5		
6		
Total:		

Date_____

Meal	Calories	Carbohydrates
1		
2		
3		
4		
5		
6		
Total:		

Date_____

Meal	Calories	Carbohydrates
1		
2		
3		
4		
5		
6		
Total:		

Date_____

Meal	Calories	Carbohydrates
1		
2		
3		
4		
5		
6		
Total:		

Date_____

Meal	Calories	Carbohydrates
1		
2		
3		
4		
5		
6		
Total:		

Date_____

Meal	Calories	Carbohydrates
1		
2		
3		
4		
5		
6		
Total:		

Date_____

Meal	Calories	Carbohydrates
1		
2		
3		
4		
5		
6		
Total:		

Date_____

Meal	Calories	Carbohydrates
1		
2		
3		
4		
5		
6		
Total:		

Date_____

Meal	Calories	Carbohydrates
1		
2		
3		
4		
5		
6		
Total:		

Date_____

Meal	Calories	Carbohydrates
1		
2		
3		
4		
5		
6		
Total:		

Date_____

Meal	Calories	Carbohydrates
1		
2		
3		
4		
5		
6		
Total:		

Date_____

Meal	Calories	Carbohydrates
1		
2		
3		
4		
5		
6		
Total:		

Date_____

Meal	Calories	Carbohydrates
1		
2		
3		
4		
5		
6		
Total:		

Date_____

Meal	Calories	Carbohydrates
1		
2		
3		
4		
5		
6		
Total:		

Date_____

Meal	Calories	Carbohydrates
1		
2		
3		
4		
5		
6		
Total:		

Date_____

Meal	Calories	Carbohydrates
1		
2		
3		
4		
5		
6		
Total:		

Date_____

Meal	Calories	Carbohydrates
1		
2		
3		
4		
5		
6		
Total:		

Date_____

Meal	Calories	Carbohydrates
1		
2		
3		
4		
5		
6		
Total:		

Date_____

Meal	Calories	Carbohydrates
1		
2		
3		
4		
5		
6		
Total:		

Date_____

Meal	Calories	Carbohydrates
1		
2		
3		
4		
5		
6		
Total:		

Date_____

Meal	Calories	Carbohydrates
1		
2		
3		
4		
5		
6		
Total:		

Date_____

Meal	Calories	Carbohydrates
1		
2		
3		
4		
5		
6		
Total:		

Date_____

Meal	Calories	Carbohydrates
1		
2		
3		
4		
5		
6		
Total:		

Date_____

Meal	Calories	Carbohydrates
1		
2		
3		
4		
5		
6		
Total:		

Date_____

Meal	Calories	Carbohydrates
1		
2		
3		
4		
5		
6		
Total:		

Date_____

Meal	Calories	Carbohydrates
1		
2		
3		
4		
5		
6		
Total:		

Date_____

Meal	Calories	Carbohydrates
1		
2		
3		
4		
5		
6		
Total:		

Date_____

Meal	Calories	Carbohydrates
1		
2		
3		
4		
5		
6		
Total:		

Date_____		
Meal	*Calories*	*Carbohydrates*
1		
2		
3		
4		
5		
6		
Total:		

Date_____		
Meal	*Calories*	*Carbohydrates*
1		
2		
3		
4		
5		
6		
Total:		

Date_____		
Meal	*Calories*	*Carbohydrates*
1		
2		
3		
4		
5		
6		
Total:		

Date_____		
Meal	*Calories*	*Carbohydrates*
1		
2		
3		
4		
5		
6		
Total:		

Date_____		
Meal	*Calories*	*Carbohydrates*
1		
2		
3		
4		
5		
6		
Total:		

Date_____		
Meal	*Calories*	*Carbohydrates*
1		
2		
3		
4		
5		
6		
Total:		

Date_____		
Meal	*Calories*	*Carbohydrates*
1		
2		
3		
4		
5		
6		
Total:		

Date_____		
Meal	*Calories*	*Carbohydrates*
1		
2		
3		
4		
5		
6		
Total:		

Date_____		
Meal	*Calories*	*Carbohydrates*
1		
2		
3		
4		
5		
6		
Total:		

Date_____		
Meal	*Calories*	*Carbohydrates*
1		
2		
3		
4		
5		
6		
Total:		

Date_____		
Meal	*Calories*	*Carbohydrates*
1		
2		
3		
4		
5		
6		
Total:		

Date_____		
Meal	*Calories*	*Carbohydrates*
1		
2		
3		
4		
5		
6		
Total:		

Date_____

Meal	Calories	Carbohydrates
1		
2		
3		
4		
5		
6		
Total:		

Date_____

Meal	Calories	Carbohydrates
1		
2		
3		
4		
5		
6		
Total:		

Date_____

Meal	Calories	Carbohydrates
1		
2		
3		
4		
5		
6		
Total:		

Date_____

Meal	Calories	Carbohydrates
1		
2		
3		
4		
5		
6		
Total:		

Date_____

Meal	Calories	Carbohydrates
1		
2		
3		
4		
5		
6		
Total:		

Date_____

Meal	Calories	Carbohydrates
1		
2		
3		
4		
5		
6		
Total:		

Date_____

Meal	Calories	Carbohydrates
1		
2		
3		
4		
5		
6		
Total:		

Date_____

Meal	Calories	Carbohydrates
1		
2		
3		
4		
5		
6		
Total:		

Date_____

Meal	Calories	Carbohydrates
1		
2		
3		
4		
5		
6		
Total:		

Date_____

Meal	Calories	Carbohydrates
1		
2		
3		
4		
5		
6		
Total:		

Date_____

Meal	Calories	Carbohydrates
1		
2		
3		
4		
5		
6		
Total:		

Date_____

Meal	Calories	Carbohydrates
1		
2		
3		
4		
5		
6		
Total:		

Date_____

Meal	Calories	Carbohydrates
1		
2		
3		
4		
5		
6		
Total:		

Date_____

Meal	Calories	Carbohydrates
1		
2		
3		
4		
5		
6		
Total:		

Date_____

Meal	Calories	Carbohydrates
1		
2		
3		
4		
5		
6		
Total:		

Date_____

Meal	Calories	Carbohydrates
1		
2		
3		
4		
5		
6		
Total:		

Date_____

Meal	Calories	Carbohydrates
1		
2		
3		
4		
5		
6		
Total:		

Date_____

Meal	Calories	Carbohydrates
1		
2		
3		
4		
5		
6		
Total:		

Date_____

Meal	Calories	Carbohydrates
1		
2		
3		
4		
5		
6		
Total:		

Date_____

Meal	Calories	Carbohydrates
1		
2		
3		
4		
5		
6		
Total:		

Date_____

Meal	Calories	Carbohydrates
1		
2		
3		
4		
5		
6		
Total:		

Date_____

Meal	Calories	Carbohydrates
1		
2		
3		
4		
5		
6		
Total:		

Date_____

Meal	Calories	Carbohydrates
1		
2		
3		
4		
5		
6		
Total:		

Date_____

Meal	Calories	Carbohydrates
1		
2		
3		
4		
5		
6		
Total:		

Date_____

Meal	Calories	Carbohydrates
1		
2		
3		
4		
5		
6		
Total:		

Date_____

Meal	Calories	Carbohydrates
1		
2		
3		
4		
5		
6		
Total:		

Date_____

Meal	Calories	Carbohydrates
1		
2		
3		
4		
5		
6		
Total:		

Date_____

Meal	Calories	Carbohydrates
1		
2		
3		
4		
5		
6		
Total:		

Date_____

Meal	Calories	Carbohydrates
1		
2		
3		
4		
5		
6		
Total:		

Date_____

Meal	Calories	Carbohydrates
1		
2		
3		
4		
5		
6		
Total:		

Date_____

Meal	Calories	Carbohydrates
1		
2		
3		
4		
5		
6		
Total:		

Date_____

Meal	Calories	Carbohydrates
1		
2		
3		
4		
5		
6		
Total:		

Date_____

Meal	Calories	Carbohydrates
1		
2		
3		
4		
5		
6		
Total:		

Date_____

Meal	Calories	Carbohydrates
1		
2		
3		
4		
5		
6		
Total:		

Date_____

Meal	Calories	Carbohydrates
1		
2		
3		
4		
5		
6		
Total:		

Date_____

Meal	Calories	Carbohydrates
1		
2		
3		
4		
5		
6		
Total:		

Date_____

Meal	Calories	Carbohydrates
1		
2		
3		
4		
5		
6		
Total:		

Date_____

Meal	Calories	Carbohydrates
1		
2		
3		
4		
5		
6		
Total:		

Date_____

Meal	Calories	Carbohydrates
1		
2		
3		
4		
5		
6		
Total:		

Date_____

Meal	Calories	Carbohydrates
1		
2		
3		
4		
5		
6		
Total:		

Date_____

Meal	Calories	Carbohydrates
1		
2		
3		
4		
5		
6		
Total:		

Date_____

Meal	Calories	Carbohydrates
1		
2		
3		
4		
5		
6		
Total:		

Date_____

Meal	Calories	Carbohydrates
1		
2		
3		
4		
5		
6		
Total:		

Date_____

Meal	Calories	Carbohydrates
1		
2		
3		
4		
5		
6		
Total:		

Date_____

Meal	Calories	Carbohydrates
1		
2		
3		
4		
5		
6		
Total:		

Date_____

Meal	Calories	Carbohydrates
1		
2		
3		
4		
5		
6		
Total:		

Date_____

Meal	Calories	Carbohydrates
1		
2		
3		
4		
5		
6		
Total:		

Date_____

Meal	Calories	Carbohydrates
1		
2		
3		
4		
5		
6		
Total:		

Date_____

Meal	Calories	Carbohydrates
1		
2		
3		
4		
5		
6		
Total:		

Date_____

Meal	Calories	Carbohydrates
1		
2		
3		
4		
5		
6		
Total:		

Date_____

Meal	Calories	Carbohydrates
1		
2		
3		
4		
5		
6		
Total:		

Date_____

Meal	Calories	Carbohydrates
1		
2		
3		
4		
5		
6		
Total:		

Date_____

Meal	Calories	Carbohydrates
1		
2		
3		
4		
5		
6		
Total:		

Date_____

Meal	Calories	Carbohydrates
1		
2		
3		
4		
5		
6		
Total:		

Date_____

Meal	Calories	Carbohydrates
1		
2		
3		
4		
5		
6		
Total:		

Date_____

Meal	Calories	Carbohydrates
1		
2		
3		
4		
5		
6		
Total:		

Date_____

Meal	Calories	Carbohydrates
1		
2		
3		
4		
5		
6		
Total:		

Date_____

Meal	Calories	Carbohydrates
1		
2		
3		
4		
5		
6		
Total:		

Date_____

Meal	Calories	Carbohydrates
1		
2		
3		
4		
5		
6		
Total:		

Date_____

Meal	Calories	Carbohydrates
1		
2		
3		
4		
5		
6		
Total:		

Date_____

Meal	Calories	Carbohydrates
1		
2		
3		
4		
5		
6		
Total:		

Date_____

Meal	Calories	Carbohydrates
1		
2		
3		
4		
5		
6		
Total:		

Date_____

Meal	Calories	Carbohydrates
1		
2		
3		
4		
5		
6		
Total:		

Date_____

Meal	Calories	Carbohydrates
1		
2		
3		
4		
5		
6		
Total:		

Date_____

Meal	Calories	Carbohydrates
1		
2		
3		
4		
5		
6		
Total:		

Date_____

Meal	Calories	Carbohydrates
1		
2		
3		
4		
5		
6		
Total:		

Date_____

Meal	Calories	Carbohydrates
1		
2		
3		
4		
5		
6		
Total:		

Date_____

Meal	Calories	Carbohydrates
1		
2		
3		
4		
5		
6		
Total:		

Date_____

Meal	Calories	Carbohydrates
1		
2		
3		
4		
5		
6		
Total:		

Date_____

Meal	Calories	Carbohydrates
1		
2		
3		
4		
5		
6		
Total:		

Date_____

Meal	Calories	Carbohydrates
1		
2		
3		
4		
5		
6		
Total:		

Date_____

Meal	Calories	Carbohydrates
1		
2		
3		
4		
5		
6		
Total:		

Date_____		
Meal	*Calories*	*Carbohydrates*
1		
2		
3		
4		
5		
6		
Total:		

Date_____		
Meal	*Calories*	*Carbohydrates*
1		
2		
3		
4		
5		
6		
Total:		

Date_____		
Meal	*Calories*	*Carbohydrates*
1		
2		
3		
4		
5		
6		
Total:		

Date_____		
Meal	*Calories*	*Carbohydrates*
1		
2		
3		
4		
5		
6		
Total:		

Date_____		
Meal	*Calories*	*Carbohydrates*
1		
2		
3		
4		
5		
6		
Total:		

Date_____		
Meal	*Calories*	*Carbohydrates*
1		
2		
3		
4		
5		
6		
Total:		

Date_____		
Meal	*Calories*	*Carbohydrates*
1		
2		
3		
4		
5		
6		
Total:		

Date_____		
Meal	*Calories*	*Carbohydrates*
1		
2		
3		
4		
5		
6		
Total:		

Date_____		
Meal	*Calories*	*Carbohydrates*
1		
2		
3		
4		
5		
6		
Total:		

Date_____		
Meal	*Calories*	*Carbohydrates*
1		
2		
3		
4		
5		
6		
Total:		

Date_____		
Meal	*Calories*	*Carbohydrates*
1		
2		
3		
4		
5		
6		
Total:		

Date_____		
Meal	*Calories*	*Carbohydrates*
1		
2		
3		
4		
5		
6		
Total:		

Date_____

Meal	Calories	Carbohydrates
1		
2		
3		
4		
5		
6		
Total:		

Date_____

Meal	Calories	Carbohydrates
1		
2		
3		
4		
5		
6		
Total:		

Date_____

Meal	Calories	Carbohydrates
1		
2		
3		
4		
5		
6		
Total:		

Date_____

Meal	Calories	Carbohydrates
1		
2		
3		
4		
5		
6		
Total:		

Date_____

Meal	Calories	Carbohydrates
1		
2		
3		
4		
5		
6		
Total:		

Date_____

Meal	Calories	Carbohydrates
1		
2		
3		
4		
5		
6		
Total:		

Date_____

Meal	Calories	Carbohydrates
1		
2		
3		
4		
5		
6		
Total:		

Date_____

Meal	Calories	Carbohydrates
1		
2		
3		
4		
5		
6		
Total:		

Date_____

Meal	Calories	Carbohydrates
1		
2		
3		
4		
5		
6		
Total:		

Date_____

Meal	Calories	Carbohydrates
1		
2		
3		
4		
5		
6		
Total:		

Date_____

Meal	Calories	Carbohydrates
1		
2		
3		
4		
5		
6		
Total:		

Date_____

Meal	Calories	Carbohydrates
1		
2		
3		
4		
5		
6		
Total:		

Date_____

Meal	Calories	Carbohydrates
1		
2		
3		
4		
5		
6		
Total:		

Date_____

Meal	Calories	Carbohydrates
1		
2		
3		
4		
5		
6		
Total:		

Date_____

Meal	Calories	Carbohydrates
1		
2		
3		
4		
5		
6		
Total:		

Date_____

Meal	Calories	Carbohydrates
1		
2		
3		
4		
5		
6		
Total:		

Date_____

Meal	Calories	Carbohydrates
1		
2		
3		
4		
5		
6		
Total:		

Date_____

Meal	Calories	Carbohydrates
1		
2		
3		
4		
5		
6		
Total:		

Date_____

Meal	Calories	Carbohydrates
1		
2		
3		
4		
5		
6		
Total:		

Date_____

Meal	Calories	Carbohydrates
1		
2		
3		
4		
5		
6		
Total:		

Date_____

Meal	Calories	Carbohydrates
1		
2		
3		
4		
5		
6		
Total:		

Date_____

Meal	Calories	Carbohydrates
1		
2		
3		
4		
5		
6		
Total:		

Date_____

Meal	Calories	Carbohydrates
1		
2		
3		
4		
5		
6		
Total:		

Date_____

Meal	Calories	Carbohydrates
1		
2		
3		
4		
5		
6		
Total:		

Date_____

Meal	Calories	Carbohydrates
1		
2		
3		
4		
5		
6		
Total:		

Date_____

Meal	Calories	Carbohydrates
1		
2		
3		
4		
5		
6		
Total:		

Date_____

Meal	Calories	Carbohydrates
1		
2		
3		
4		
5		
6		
Total:		

Date_____

Meal	Calories	Carbohydrates
1		
2		
3		
4		
5		
6		
Total:		

Date_____

Meal	Calories	Carbohydrates
1		
2		
3		
4		
5		
6		
Total:		

Date_____

Meal	Calories	Carbohydrates
1		
2		
3		
4		
5		
6		
Total:		

Date_____

Meal	Calories	Carbohydrates
1		
2		
3		
4		
5		
6		
Total:		

Date_____

Meal	Calories	Carbohydrates
1		
2		
3		
4		
5		
6		
Total:		

Date_____

Meal	Calories	Carbohydrates
1		
2		
3		
4		
5		
6		
Total:		

Date_____

Meal	Calories	Carbohydrates
1		
2		
3		
4		
5		
6		
Total:		

Date_____

Meal	Calories	Carbohydrates
1		
2		
3		
4		
5		
6		
Total:		

Date_____

Meal	Calories	Carbohydrates
1		
2		
3		
4		
5		
6		
Total:		

Date_____

Meal	Calories	Carbohydrates
1		
2		
3		
4		
5		
6		
Total:		

Date_____

Meal	Calories	Carbohydrates
1		
2		
3		
4		
5		
6		
Total:		

Date_____

Meal	Calories	Carbohydrates
1		
2		
3		
4		
5		
6		
Total:		

Date_____

Meal	Calories	Carbohydrates
1		
2		
3		
4		
5		
6		
Total:		

Date_____

Meal	Calories	Carbohydrates
1		
2		
3		
4		
5		
6		
Total:		

Date_____

Meal	Calories	Carbohydrates
1		
2		
3		
4		
5		
6		
Total:		

Date_____

Meal	Calories	Carbohydrates
1		
2		
3		
4		
5		
6		
Total:		

Date_____

Meal	Calories	Carbohydrates
1		
2		
3		
4		
5		
6		
Total:		

Date_____

Meal	Calories	Carbohydrates
1		
2		
3		
4		
5		
6		
Total:		

Date_____

Meal	Calories	Carbohydrates
1		
2		
3		
4		
5		
6		
Total:		

Date_____

Meal	Calories	Carbohydrates
1		
2		
3		
4		
5		
6		
Total:		

Date_____

Meal	Calories	Carbohydrates
1		
2		
3		
4		
5		
6		
Total:		

Date_____

Meal	Calories	Carbohydrates
1		
2		
3		
4		
5		
6		
Total:		

Date_____

Meal	Calories	Carbohydrates
1		
2		
3		
4		
5		
6		
Total:		

Date_____

Meal	Calories	Carbohydrates
1		
2		
3		
4		
5		
6		
Total:		

Date_____

Meal	Calories	Carbohydrates
1		
2		
3		
4		
5		
6		
Total:		

Date_____

Meal	Calories	Carbohydrates
1		
2		
3		
4		
5		
6		
Total:		

Date_____

Meal	Calories	Carbohydrates
1		
2		
3		
4		
5		
6		
Total:		

Date_____

Meal	Calories	Carbohydrates
1		
2		
3		
4		
5		
6		
Total:		

Date_____

Meal	Calories	Carbohydrates
1		
2		
3		
4		
5		
6		
Total:		

Date_____

Meal	Calories	Carbohydrates
1		
2		
3		
4		
5		
6		
Total:		

Date_____

Meal	Calories	Carbohydrates
1		
2		
3		
4		
5		
6		
Total:		

Date_____

Meal	Calories	Carbohydrates
1		
2		
3		
4		
5		
6		
Total:		

Date_____

Meal	Calories	Carbohydrates
1		
2		
3		
4		
5		
6		
Total:		

Date_____

Meal	Calories	Carbohydrates
1		
2		
3		
4		
5		
6		
Total:		

Date_____

Meal	Calories	Carbohydrates
1		
2		
3		
4		
5		
6		
Total:		

Date_____

Meal	Calories	Carbohydrates
1		
2		
3		
4		
5		
6		
Total:		

Date_____

Meal	Calories	Carbohydrates
1		
2		
3		
4		
5		
6		
Total:		

Date_____

Meal	Calories	Carbohydrates
1		
2		
3		
4		
5		
6		
Total:		

Date_____

Meal	Calories	Carbohydrates
1		
2		
3		
4		
5		
6		
Total:		

Date_____

Meal	Calories	Carbohydrates
1		
2		
3		
4		
5		
6		
Total:		

Date_____

Meal	Calories	Carbohydrates
1		
2		
3		
4		
5		
6		
Total:		

Date_____

Meal	Calories	Carbohydrates
1		
2		
3		
4		
5		
6		
Total:		

Date_____

Meal	Calories	Carbohydrates
1		
2		
3		
4		
5		
6		
Total:		

Date_____

Meal	Calories	Carbohydrates
1		
2		
3		
4		
5		
6		
Total:		

Date_____

Meal	Calories	Carbohydrates
1		
2		
3		
4		
5		
6		
Total:		

Date_____

Meal	Calories	Carbohydrates
1		
2		
3		
4		
5		
6		
Total:		

Date_____

Meal	Calories	Carbohydrates
1		
2		
3		
4		
5		
6		
Total:		

Date_____

Meal	Calories	Carbohydrates
1		
2		
3		
4		
5		
6		
Total:		

Date_____

Meal	Calories	Carbohydrates
1		
2		
3		
4		
5		
6		
Total:		

Date_____

Meal	Calories	Carbohydrates
1		
2		
3		
4		
5		
6		
Total:		

Date_____

Meal	Calories	Carbohydrates
1		
2		
3		
4		
5		
6		
Total:		

Date_____

Meal	Calories	Carbohydrates
1		
2		
3		
4		
5		
6		
Total:		

Date_____

Meal	Calories	Carbohydrates
1		
2		
3		
4		
5		
6		
Total:		

Date_____

Meal	Calories	Carbohydrates
1		
2		
3		
4		
5		
6		
Total:		

Date_____

Meal	Calories	Carbohydrates
1		
2		
3		
4		
5		
6		
Total:		

Date_____

Meal	Calories	Carbohydrates
1		
2		
3		
4		
5		
6		
Total:		

Date_____

Meal	Calories	Carbohydrates
1		
2		
3		
4		
5		
6		
Total:		

Date_____

Meal	Calories	Carbohydrates
1		
2		
3		
4		
5		
6		
Total:		

Date_____

Meal	Calories	Carbohydrates
1		
2		
3		
4		
5		
6		
Total:		

Date_____

Meal	Calories	Carbohydrates
1		
2		
3		
4		
5		
6		
Total:		

Date_____

Meal	Calories	Carbohydrates
1		
2		
3		
4		
5		
6		
Total:		

Date_____

Meal	Calories	Carbohydrates
1		
2		
3		
4		
5		
6		
Total:		

Date_____

Meal	Calories	Carbohydrates
1		
2		
3		
4		
5		
6		
Total:		

Date_____

Meal	Calories	Carbohydrates
1		
2		
3		
4		
5		
6		
Total:		

Date_____

Meal	Calories	Carbohydrates
1		
2		
3		
4		
5		
6		
Total:		

Date_____

Meal	Calories	Carbohydrates
1		
2		
3		
4		
5		
6		
Total:		

Date_____

Meal	Calories	Carbohydrates
1		
2		
3		
4		
5		
6		
Total:		

Date_____

Meal	Calories	Carbohydrates
1		
2		
3		
4		
5		
6		
Total:		

Date_____

Meal	Calories	Carbohydrates
1		
2		
3		
4		
5		
6		
Total:		

Date_____

Meal	Calories	Carbohydrates
1		
2		
3		
4		
5		
6		
Total:		

Date_____

Meal	Calories	Carbohydrates
1		
2		
3		
4		
5		
6		
Total:		

Date_____

Meal	Calories	Carbohydrates
1		
2		
3		
4		
5		
6		
Total:		

Date_____

Meal	Calories	Carbohydrates
1		
2		
3		
4		
5		
6		
Total:		

Date_____

Meal	Calories	Carbohydrates
1		
2		
3		
4		
5		
6		
Total:		

Date_____

Meal	Calories	Carbohydrates
1		
2		
3		
4		
5		
6		
Total:		

Date_____

Meal	Calories	Carbohydrates
1		
2		
3		
4		
5		
6		
Total:		

Date_____

Meal	Calories	Carbohydrates
1		
2		
3		
4		
5		
6		
Total:		

Date_____

Meal	Calories	Carbohydrates
1		
2		
3		
4		
5		
6		
Total:		

Date_____

Meal	Calories	Carbohydrates
1		
2		
3		
4		
5		
6		
Total:		

Date_____

Meal	Calories	Carbohydrates
1		
2		
3		
4		
5		
6		
Total:		

Date_____

Meal	Calories	Carbohydrates
1		
2		
3		
4		
5		
6		
Total:		

Date_____

Meal	Calories	Carbohydrates
1		
2		
3		
4		
5		
6		
Total:		

Date_____

Meal	Calories	Carbohydrates
1		
2		
3		
4		
5		
6		
Total:		

Date_____

Meal	Calories	Carbohydrates
1		
2		
3		
4		
5		
6		
Total:		

Date_____

Meal	Calories	Carbohydrates
1		
2		
3		
4		
5		
6		
Total:		

Date_____

Meal	Calories	Carbohydrates
1		
2		
3		
4		
5		
6		
Total:		

Date_____

Meal	Calories	Carbohydrates
1		
2		
3		
4		
5		
6		
Total:		

	Calories	Carbohydrates
1		
2		
3		
4		
5		
6		
Total:		

Date_____

Meal	Calories	Carbohydrates
1		
2		
3		
4		
5		
6		
Total:		

Date_____

Meal	Calories	Carbohydrates
1		
2		
3		
4		
5		
6		
Total:		

Date_____

Meal	Calories	Carbohydrates
1		
2		
3		
4		
5		
6		
Total:		

ate_____

Meal	Calories	Carbohydrates
1		
2		
3		
4		
5		
6		
Total:		

Date_____

Meal	Calories	Carbohydrates
1		
2		
3		
4		
5		
6		
Total:		

Date_____

Meal	Calories	Carbohydrates
1		
2		
3		
4		
5		
6		
Total:		

Date_____

Meal	Calories	Carbohydrates
1		
2		
3		
4		
5		
6		
Total:		

Date_____

Meal	Calories	Carbohydrates
1		
2		
3		
4		
5		
6		
Total:		

Date_____

Meal	Calories	Carbohydrates
1		
2		
3		
4		
5		
6		
Total:		

Date_____

Meal	Calories	Carbohydrates
1		
2		
3		
4		
5		
6		
Total:		

Date_____

Meal	Calories	Carbohydrates
1		
2		
3		
4		
5		
6		
Total:		

Date		
Meal	*Calories*	*Carbohydrates*
1		
2		
3		
4		
5		
6		
Total:		

Date		
Meal	*Calories*	*Carbohydrates*
1		
2		
3		
4		
5		
6		
Total:		

Date		
Meal	*Calories*	*Carbohydrates*
1		
2		
3		
4		
5		
6		
Total:		

Date	
Meal	*Calories*
1	
2	
3	
4	
5	
6	
Total:	

Date		
Meal	*Calories*	*Carbohydrates*
1		
2		
3		
4		
5		
6		
Total:		

Date		
Meal	*Calories*	*Carbohydrates*
1		
2		
3		
4		
5		
6		
Total:		

Date		
Meal	*Calories*	*Carbohydrates*
1		
2		
3		
4		
5		
6		
Total:		

Date		
Meal	*Calories*	*Ca*
1		
2		
3		
4		
5		
6		
Total:		

Date		
Meal	*Calories*	*Carbohydrates*
1		
2		
3		
4		
5		
6		
Total:		

Date		
Meal	*Calories*	*Carbohydrates*
1		
2		
3		
4		
5		
6		
Total:		

Date		
Meal	*Calories*	*Carbohydrates*
1		
2		
3		
4		
5		
6		
Total:		

Date		
Meal	*Calories*	*Carbohydrates*
1		
2		
3		
4		
5		
6		
Total:		

Date_____

Meal	Calories	Carbohydrates
1		
2		
3		
4		
5		
6		
Total:		

Date_____

Meal	Calories	Carbohydrates
1		
2		
3		
4		
5		
6		
Total:		

Date_____

Meal	Calories	Carbohydrates
1		
2		
3		
4		
5		
6		
Total:		

Date_____

Meal	Calories	Carbohydrates
1		
2		
3		
4		
5		
6		
Total:		

Date_____

Meal	Calories	Carbohydrates
1		
2		
3		
4		
5		
6		
Total:		

Date_____

Meal	Calories	Carbohydrates
1		
2		
3		
4		
5		
6		
Total:		

Date_____

Meal	Calories	Carbohydrates
1		
2		
3		
4		
5		
6		
Total:		

Date_____

Meal	Calories	Carbohydrates
1		
2		
3		
4		
5		
6		
Total:		

Date_____

Meal	Calories	Carbohydrates
1		
2		
3		
4		
5		
6		
Total:		

Date_____

Meal	Calories	Carbohydrates
1		
2		
3		
4		
5		
6		
Total:		

Date_____

Meal	Calories	Carbohydrates
1		
2		
3		
4		
5		
6		
Total:		

Date_____

Meal	Calories	Carbohydrates
1		
2		
3		
4		
5		
6		
Total:		

Date_____

Meal	Calories	Carbohydrates
1		
2		
3		
4		
5		
6		
Total:		

Date_____

Meal	Calories	Carbohydrates
1		
2		
3		
4		
5		
6		
Total:		

Date_____

Meal	Calories	Carbohydrates
1		
2		
3		
4		
5		
6		
Total:		

Date_____

Meal	Calories	Carbohydrates
1		
2		
3		
4		
5		
6		
Total:		

Date_____

Meal	Calories	Carbohydrates
1		
2		
3		
4		
5		
6		
Total:		

Date_____

Meal	Calories	Carbohydrates
1		
2		
3		
4		
5		
6		
Total:		

Date_____		
Meal	*Calories*	*Carbohydrates*
1		
2		
3		
4		
5		
6		
Total:		

Date_____		
Meal	*Calories*	*Carbohydrates*
1		
2		
3		
4		
5		
6		
Total:		

Date_____		
Meal	*Calories*	*Carbohydrates*
1		
2		
3		
4		
5		
6		
Total:		

Date_____		
Meal	*Calories*	*Carbohydrates*
1		
2		
3		
4		
5		
6		
Total:		

Date_____		
Meal	*Calories*	*Carbohydrates*
1		
2		
3		
4		
5		
6		
Total:		

Date_____		
Meal	*Calories*	*Carbohydrates*
1		
2		
3		
4		
5		
6		
Total:		

Date_____

Meal	Calories	Carbohydrates
1		
2		
3		
4		
5		
6		
Total:		

Date_____

Meal	Calories	Carbohydrates
1		
2		
3		
4		
5		
6		
Total:		

Date_____

Meal	Calories	Carbohydrates
1		
2		
3		
4		
5		
6		
Total:		

Date_____

Meal	Calories	Carbohydrates
1		
2		
3		
4		
5		
6		
Total:		

Date_____

Meal	Calories	Carbohydrates
1		
2		
3		
4		
5		
6		
Total:		

Date_____

Meal	Calories	Carbohydrates
1		
2		
3		
4		
5		
6		
Total:		

Date_____

Meal	Calories	Carbohydrates
1		
2		
3		
4		
5		
6		
Total:		

Date_____

Meal	Calories	Carbohydrates
1		
2		
3		
4		
5		
6		
Total:		

Date_____

Meal	Calories	Carbohydrates
1		
2		
3		
4		
5		
6		
Total:		

Date_____

Meal	Calories	Carbohydrates
1		
2		
3		
4		
5		
6		
Total:		

Date_____

Meal	Calories	Carbohydrates
1		
2		
3		
4		
5		
6		
Total:		

Date_____

Meal	Calories	Carbohydrates
1		
2		
3		
4		
5		
6		
Total:		

Date_____

Meal	Calories	Carbohydrates
1		
2		
3		
4		
5		
6		
Total:		

Date_____

Meal	Calories	Carbohydrates
1		
2		
3		
4		
5		
6		
Total:		

Date_____

Meal	Calories	Carbohydrates
1		
2		
3		
4		
5		
6		
Total:		

Date_____

Meal	Calories	Carbohydrates
1		
2		
3		
4		
5		
6		
Total:		

Date_____

Meal	Calories	Carbohydrates
1		
2		
3		
4		
5		
6		
Total:		

Date_____

Meal	Calories	Carbohydrates
1		
2		
3		
4		
5		
6		
Total:		

Date_____

Meal	Calories	Carbohydrates
1		
2		
3		
4		
5		
6		
Total:		

Date_____

Meal	Calories	Carbohydrates
1		
2		
3		
4		
5		
6		
Total:		

Date_____

Meal	Calories	Carbohydrates
1		
2		
3		
4		
5		
6		
Total:		

Date_____

Meal	Calories	Carbohydrates
1		
2		
3		
4		
5		
6		
Total:		

Date_____

Meal	Calories	Carbohydrates
1		
2		
3		
4		
5		
6		
Total:		

Date_____

Meal	Calories	Carbohydrates
1		
2		
3		
4		
5		
6		
Total:		

Date_____

Meal	Calories	Carbohydrates
1		
2		
3		
4		
5		
6		
Total:		

Date_____

Meal	Calories	Carbohydrates
1		
2		
3		
4		
5		
6		
Total:		

Date_____

Meal	Calories	Carbohydrates
1		
2		
3		
4		
5		
6		
Total:		

Date_____

Meal	Calories	Carbohydrates
1		
2		
3		
4		
5		
6		
Total:		

Date_____

Meal	Calories	Carbohydrates
1		
2		
3		
4		
5		
6		
Total:		

Date_____

Meal	Calories	Carbohydrates
1		
2		
3		
4		
5		
6		
Total:		

Date_____

Meal	Calories	Carbohydrates
1		
2		
3		
4		
5		
6		
Total:		

Date_____

Meal	Calories	Carbohydrates
1		
2		
3		
4		
5		
6		
Total:		

Date_____

Meal	Calories	Carbohydrates
1		
2		
3		
4		
5		
6		
Total:		

Date_____

Meal	Calories	Carbohydrates
1		
2		
3		
4		
5		
6		
Total:		

Date_____

Meal	Calories	Carbohydrates
1		
2		
3		
4		
5		
6		
Total:		

Date_____

Meal	Calories	Carbohydrates
1		
2		
3		
4		
5		
6		
Total:		

Date_____

Meal	Calories	Carbohydrates
1		
2		
3		
4		
5		
6		
Total:		

Date_____

Meal	Calories	Carbohydrates
1		
2		
3		
4		
5		
6		
Total:		

Date_____

Meal	Calories	Carbohydrates
1		
2		
3		
4		
5		
6		
Total:		

Date_____

Meal	Calories	Carbohydrates
1		
2		
3		
4		
5		
6		
Total:		

Date_____

Meal	Calories	Carbohydrates
1		
2		
3		
4		
5		
6		
Total:		

Date_____

Meal	Calories	Carbohydrates
1		
2		
3		
4		
5		
6		
Total:		

Date_____

Meal	Calories	Carbohydrates
1		
2		
3		
4		
5		
6		
Total:		

Date_____

Meal	Calories	Carbohydrates
1		
2		
3		
4		
5		
6		
Total:		

Date_____

Meal	Calories	Carbohydrates
1		
2		
3		
4		
5		
6		
Total:		

Date_____

Meal	Calories	Carbohydrates
1		
2		
3		
4		
5		
6		
Total:		

Date_____

Meal	Calories	Carbohydrates
1		
2		
3		
4		
5		
6		
Total:		

Date_____

Meal	Calories	Carbohydrates
1		
2		
3		
4		
5		
6		
Total:		

Date_____

Meal	Calories	Carbohydrates
1		
2		
3		
4		
5		
6		
Total:		

Date_____

Meal	Calories	Carbohydrates
1		
2		
3		
4		
5		
6		
Total:		

Date_____

Meal	Calories	Carbohydrates
1		
2		
3		
4		
5		
6		
Total:		

Date_____

Meal	Calories	Carbohydrates
1		
2		
3		
4		
5		
6		
Total:		

Date_____

Meal	Calories	Carbohydrates
1		
2		
3		
4		
5		
6		
Total:		

Date_____

Meal	Calories	Carbohydrates
1		
2		
3		
4		
5		
6		
Total:		

Date_____

Meal	Calories	Carbohydrates
1		
2		
3		
4		
5		
6		
Total:		

Date_____

Meal	Calories	Carbohydrates
1		
2		
3		
4		
5		
6		
Total:		

Date_____

Meal	Calories	Carbohydrates
1		
2		
3		
4		
5		
6		
Total:		

Date_____

Meal	Calories	Carbohydrates
1		
2		
3		
4		
5		
6		
Total:		

Date_____

Meal	Calories	Carbohydrates
1		
2		
3		
4		
5		
6		
Total:		

Date_____

Meal	Calories	Carbohydrates
1		
2		
3		
4		
5		
6		
Total:		

Date_____

Meal	Calories	Carbohydrates
1		
2		
3		
4		
5		
6		
Total:		

Date_____

Meal	Calories	Carbohydrates
1		
2		
3		
4		
5		
6		
Total:		

Date_____

Meal	Calories	Carbohydrates
1		
2		
3		
4		
5		
6		
Total:		

Date_____

Meal	Calories	Carbohydrates
1		
2		
3		
4		
5		
6		
Total:		

Date_____

Meal	Calories	Carbohydrates
1		
2		
3		
4		
5		
6		
Total:		

Date_____

Meal	Calories	Carbohydrates
1		
2		
3		
4		
5		
6		
Total:		

Date_____

Meal	Calories	Carbohydrates
1		
2		
3		
4		
5		
6		
Total:		

Date_____

Meal	Calories	Carbohydrates
1		
2		
3		
4		
5		
6		
Total:		

Date_____

Meal	Calories	Carbohydrates
1		
2		
3		
4		
5		
6		
Total:		

Date_____

Meal	Calories	Carbohydrates
1		
2		
3		
4		
5		
6		
Total:		

Date_____

Meal	Calories	Carbohydrates
1		
2		
3		
4		
5		
6		
Total:		

Date_____

Meal	Calories	Carbohydrates
1		
2		
3		
4		
5		
6		
Total:		

Date_____

Meal	Calories	Carbohydrates
1		
2		
3		
4		
5		
6		
Total:		

Date_____

Meal	Calories	Carbohydrates
1		
2		
3		
4		
5		
6		
Total:		

Date_____

Meal	Calories	Carbohydrates
1		
2		
3		
4		
5		
6		
Total:		

Date_____

Meal	Calories	Carbohydrates
1		
2		
3		
4		
5		
6		
Total:		

Date_____

Meal	Calories	Carbohydrates
1		
2		
3		
4		
5		
6		
Total:		

Date_____

Meal	Calories	Carbohydrates
1		
2		
3		
4		
5		
6		
Total:		

Date_____

Meal	Calories	Carbohydrates
1		
2		
3		
4		
5		
6		
Total:		

Date_____

Meal	Calories	Carbohydrates
1		
2		
3		
4		
5		
6		
Total:		

Date_____

Meal	Calories	Carbohydrates
1		
2		
3		
4		
5		
6		
Total:		

Date_____

Meal	Calories	Carbohydrates
1		
2		
3		
4		
5		
6		
Total:		

Date_____

Meal	Calories	Carbohydrates
1		
2		
3		
4		
5		
6		
Total:		

Date_____

Meal	Calories	Carbohydrates
1		
2		
3		
4		
5		
6		
Total:		

Date_____

Meal	Calories	Carbohydrates
1		
2		
3		
4		
5		
6		
Total:		

Date_____

Meal	Calories	Carbohydrates
1		
2		
3		
4		
5		
6		
Total:		

Date_____

Meal	Calories	Carbohydrates
1		
2		
3		
4		
5		
6		
Total:		

Date_____

Meal	Calories	Carbohydrates
1		
2		
3		
4		
5		
6		
Total:		

Date_____

Meal	Calories	Carbohydrates
1		
2		
3		
4		
5		
6		
Total:		

Date_____

Meal	Calories	Carbohydrates
1		
2		
3		
4		
5		
6		
Total:		

PHASE 3. RETRAINING YOUR METABOLISM

SAMPLE CHART

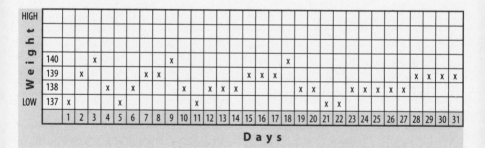

Weight	1	2	3	4	5	6	7	8	9	10	11	12	13	14	15	16	17	18	19	20	21	22	23	24	25	26	27	28	29	30	31
HIGH																															
140			x					x									x														
139		x				x	x							x	x	x												x	x	x	x
138				x		x			x		x	x	x						x	x			x	x	x	x	x				
LOW 137	x				x					x											x	x									

Days

our low weight is 137. Your high weight is 140. Keep track of your weight every day on the Phase 3 chart. Use a new chart for each month. You can eat normally until you reach your high weight (140), which, in this sample Phase 3 chart, occurs on Day 3. When you reach your high weight, go back on Phase 1 until you get down to your low weight (137), which happens here on Day 5. From Day 5, you can eat normally until you reach your high weight (140), which happens here on Day 9. When you reach your high weight, go back on Phase 1 until you reach your low weight (137), which happens here on Day 11.

From Day 11, you can eat normally until Day 18, when you hit your high weight (140) and must go back on Phase 1. Stay on Phase 1 until you reach your low weight (137) on Day 21. From Days 21 to 31, you are eating normally. If you were following this sample chart, you would be eating normally until the next time you hit your high weight of 140. Notice that each time you cycle in and out of Phase 1, you are able to eat normally for a longer period of time before you have to go back on Phase 1. Why? Your metabolism is increasing as your body rids itself of its starvation hormones.

You can photocopy additional charts directly from this book, or you can download them from my website:

www.curvesinternational.com.

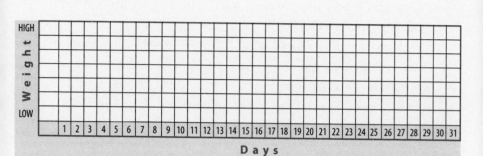

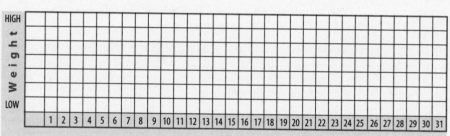

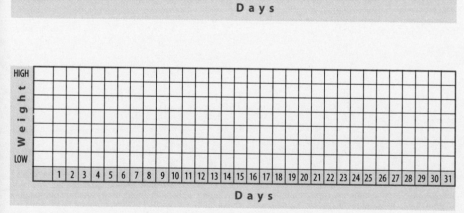

THE METABOLIC
TUNE-UP CHART

SAMPLE CHART

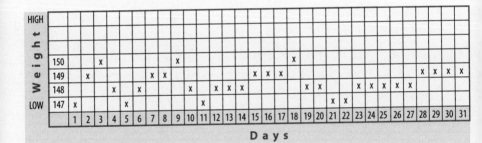

Your current weight (your low weight) is 147. Your high weight is 150. Keep track of your weight every day on the Phase 3 chart. Use a new chart for each month. You can eat normally until you reach your high weight (150), which, in this sample Phase 3 chart, occurs on Day 3. When you reach your high weight, go back on Phase 1 until you get down to your low weight (147), which happens here on

Day 5. From Day 5, you can eat normally until you reach your high weight (150), which happens here on Day 9. When you reach your high weight, go back on Phase 1 until you reach your low weight (147), which happens here on Day 11.

From Day 11, you can eat normally until Day 18, when you hit your high weight (150) and must go back on Phase 1. Stay on Phase 1 until you reach your low weight (147), which happens here on Day 21. From Day 21, you are eating normally. If you were following this sample chart, you would eat normally until the next time you hit your high weight of 150. Notice that each time you cycle in and out of Phase 1 you are able to eat normally for a longer period of time before you have to go back on Phase 1. Why? Your metabolism is increasing as your body rids itself of its starvation hormones.

When you are able to go for three to four weeks at a time without gaining weight, you are ready to resume your weight-loss program.

You can photocopy additional charts directly from this book, or you can download them from my website, www.curvesinternational.com.

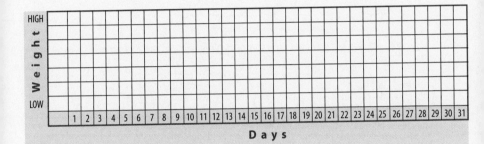

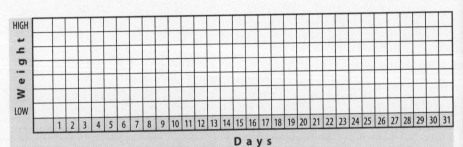

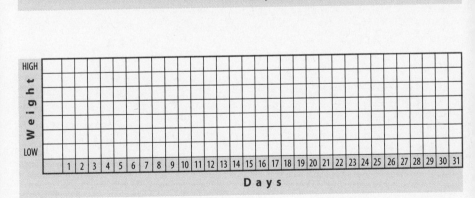

MEASUREMENT CHART

KEEPING TRACK OF YOUR PROGRESS IS IMPORTANT.

WEEK 1
Beginning Measurements

Bust _____

Waist _____

Abdomen _____

Hip _____

Thigh _____

Calf _____

Arm _____

Weight _____

Body Fat % _____

Fat lbs. _____

Date _____

WEEK 4
Measurements

Bust _____

Waist _____

Abdomen _____

Hip _____

Thigh _____

Calf _____

Arm _____

Weight _____

Body Fat % _____

Fat lbs. _____

Date _____

WEEK 6
Ending Measurements

Bust _____

Waist _____

Abdomen _____

Hip _____

Thigh _____

Calf _____

Arm _____

Weight _____

Body Fat % _____

Fat lbs. _____

Date _____

GOAL
Measurements

Bust _____

Waist _____

Abdomen _____

Hip _____

Thigh _____

Calf _____

Arm _____

Weight _____

Body Fat % _____

Fat lbs. _____

Date _____

PART FIVE

The Healthy Woman

MENOPAUSE:
A HEALTHY ALTERNATIVE

Having trouble sleeping? Tired of those extra inches around your waistline? Or maybe you're just feeling worn out and tired? If you're a forty-something woman, you are probably experiencing at least some of the classic symptoms of menopause, including the infamous hot flashes, insomnia, depression, memory problems, weight creep, and irritability. For up to a full decade before and after the cessation of your last period, your body undergoes hormonal changes that can affect your weight, your mood, and your health. Menopause also puts you at increased risk of heart disease, the number one killer of women, and osteoporosis (the thinning of your bones), which makes you vulnerable to bone fractures.

Until recently, millions of women took hormone replacement therapy (HRT) to control symptoms of menopause, and to preserve bone under the mistaken impression that it would protect their hearts. The Women's Health Initiative, a major study involving sixteen thousand women on HRT, recently reported that women who took a combination estrogen–synthetic progestin pill for more than five years were at 29 percent greater risk of having a heart attack than women taking a placebo and a 40 percent greater risk for stroke. Moreover, women who had taken HRT for more than five years were at a 26 percent increased risk of developing breast cancer. The only positive findings for HRT are (1) it helps relieve symptoms of menopause such as hot flashes and (2) it appears to protect against bone loss. Now that recent studies have revealed that hormone replacement therapy can be risky to your health, many women have stopped taking HRT, but that doesn't mean that you have to resign yourself to living a lesser life. There are healthier, more effective ways to relieve your symptoms and protect against bone loss.

SUPPLEMENTS TO RELIEVE SYMPTOMS

There are several nutritional supplements that can reduce menopausal symptoms and improve your physical and mental well-being. They can be purchased separately, or found in combination formulas specially designed for menopausal women. One popular herb, Black Cohosh, is particularly helpful in relieving hot flashes, and is medically approved for this use in Germany, a country that takes herbal medicine very seriously. Black cohosh has been around for a long time. Your great-great-grandmother probably used it in her day. (If you're suffering from menopausal symptoms, try Curves Herbal FEM; it's our unique herbal blend designed to maintain a woman's biochemistry during this transitional period.) Plant estrogens found in soy-based products (like the Curves shake, tofu, and tempeh is made from soy protein) can also help relieve mild menopausal symptoms. The worst symptoms of menopause typically pass within the first year, and many women find that these natural remedies can help ease them through that difficult period until their biochemistry normalizes.

THE RIGHT CALCIUM

Once a woman reaches menopause, she needs to take 1,500 mg. of calcium daily to preserve her bone. There are many different types of calcium on the market, and not all of them are equally effective. Calcium citrate and calcium malate are the forms of calcium that are best absorbed by the body. Moreover, according to a study conducted at the University of California, when combined with 400 IU of vitamin D and the right minerals, this special combination of calcium has been shown to *increase* bone mass in postmenopausal women. No other form of calcium has ever been shown to increase bone mass. Not even estrogen can increase bone mass: it can prevent bone loss, but it doesn't make new bone! When I read about this study, I decided to use this type of calcium in Curves Essential, our special formula for bone health. I don't think that women should settle for anything less.

THE FITNESS PRESCRIPTION

The good news is, embarking on a fitness program can be powerful preventive medicine to ease you through menopause. The even better news is that simply exercising for thirty minutes, three times a week, is all it takes to turn the odds in your favor.

- Women who engage in regular physical activity report fewer unpleasant menopausal symptoms than sedentary women.
- According to the Centers for Disease Control in Atlanta, regular physical exercise decreases your risk of colon cancer, heart disease, diabetes, and high blood pressure.

- Muscle tissue burns more calories than fat tissue: A pound of muscle burns 50 calories per day at rest; a pound of fat burns almost no calories. The bottom line is, more muscle = a leaner and trimmer body at any age.
- Weight-bearing exercise (strength training with weights, walking, running, working out on machines) maintains and strengthens bone density.
- No more hot flashes! Women who exercise regularly have fewer hot flashes than women who don't.
- Exercise can relieve depression as well or even better than antidepressants, with absolutely no side effects. It is also a great stress reliever.
- Exercise can help preserve joint health, which can prevent or reduce the symptoms of arthritis.
- Regular exercise is good for your brain, and can help maintain memory and cognitive function.
- One hour of moderate activity each day (that includes walking to the bus stop instead of driving, climbing stairs instead of taking the elevator, running errands on foot, or working out) can cut your risk of type 2 diabetes (adult-onset diabetes) by half. Type 2 diabetes increases your risk of heart attack and stroke.
- Having a fit and strong body gives you a feeling of well-being and confidence.

WHAT WOMEN NEED TO KNOW ABOUT HEART DISEASE

Although many women tend to think of heart disease as a man's problem, in reality, more than 250,000 women die of diseases of the heart and blood vessels each year. Most cases of heart disease are caused by atherosclerosis, which occurs when the arteries delivering blood and oxygen to the heart become clogged with a waxy-like substance called plaque. Plaque consists of a variety of cells, including cholesterol, a fat or lipid produced by the liver. A heart attack can occur when the arteries become so filled with plaque that it blocks the flow of blood and oxygen to the heart, which can damage and even kill significant portions of the heart.

Although heart disease may affect men at a younger age, after menopause, a woman's risk of having a heart attack increases with each passing year. Ten years after menopause, women and men are at equal risk of having a heart attack. What's unequal is the fact that women are more likely to die from their first attack than men. Half of all women die of their first attack, as opposed to one out of four men.

One of the problems is that women may not seek medical help until their hearts have suffered significant damage. Shockingly, more than one-third of all heart attacks in women go unnoticed or unreported! Many women suffer from so-called silent heart attacks; that is, the symptoms are so subtle that they are unaware they are having a heart attack. Moreover, women often have different symptoms when they are having a heart attack than men, and may not have the telltale chest pain. Every woman should know the warning signs of a heart attack. It could save her life, or the life of a loved one.

SYMPTOMS OF A HEART ATTACK COMMON TO MEN AND WOMEN

- Intense pressure or crushing pain in your chest that may radiate to your shoulder, neck, back, or jaw.
- Pounding of the heart or heart palpitations.
- Difficulty breathing, feeling unable to catch your breath, or shortness of breath.
- Nausea, vomiting, or intense indigestion that doesn't go away after taking an antacid.
- Dizziness or feeling light-headed.
- A feeling of impending doom or extreme anxiety.

WOMEN: TAKE NOTE

The following symptoms affect primarily women, and are often ignored or overlooked, even by health care practitioners:

- Sudden onset of body aches, weakness, flu-like symptoms.

- A mild sensation of burning in the chest typically dismissed as "heartburn" or indigestion that doesn't go away after taking antacids.
- Mild discomfort or ache in the chest or back.

If you think you are having a heart attack, call 911 and call your doctor to get immediate medical attention. If you are convinced that you or a loved one is having a heart attack, don't be put off by emergency room personnel who may still be under the mistaken belief that heart disease is not a woman's problem. Unfortunately, several studies have shown that a woman is less likely than a man to get prompt treatment for a heart attack, even if she seeks medical help. Women's health advocacy groups recommend that any woman who believes she is having a heart attack should insist on having an EKG and an enzyme test to get a definitive diagnosis. Work out an emergency plan with your doctor ahead of time, and make sure your family members are aware of who to call and where to go if you or any member of the family needs emergency care.

SYMPTOMS OF STROKE

hirty minutes of moderate exercise daily can reduce your risk of stroke by 20 percent.

Stroke is the third leading cause of death in women. Twice as many women die of stroke than of breast cancer! A stroke is often called a brain attack because, similar to a heart attack, the most common cause of stroke is a blockage of an artery, interrupting blood flow to a part of the brain.

The ideal approach to stroke is prevention—that is, reducing or eliminating important risk factors. High blood pressure, high cholesterol and triglycerides, smoking, diabetes, obesity, excessive alcohol intake (more than two drinks daily), and a sedentary lifestyle are among the well-known risk factors for both stroke and heart disease. Women who take estrogen—either in the form of oral contraceptives or hormone replacement therapy—are also at greater risk. The risk of stroke greatly increases if you are taking hormones and you smoke (a very bad idea).

Many people are unaware of the warning signs of stroke, and therefore don't seek immediate medical help. Prompt medical intervention can help prevent or reduce long-term damage to your brain, which can have a significant affect on quality of life.

If you have any of the symptoms listed below, call 911 for emergency care. Don't try to drive yourself to the hospital, even if you think you can.

- Unexplained dizziness or feelings of unsteadiness
- Loss of vision, especially in one eye
- Loss of speech, or difficulty talking or understanding speech
- Any unexplained weakness or numbness in the face, arms, legs, or on one side of the body.
- A severe headache unlike anything you have experienced before.

People may experience one or more of these symptoms very briefly and then resume normal activity. This is called a transient ischemic attack, or TIA. It is common to have several TIAs before having a full-blown stroke. Don't ignore a TIA. It is potentially very serious and you must get immediate medical attention.

ABOUT THE AUTHORS

Twenty-eight years ago, at the age of twenty, Gary Heavin began his career as a nutrition counselor and fitness instructor. Over the years, he has personally coached thousands of women through the process of attaining optimal weight and health. He and his wife, Diane, perfected the Curves concept at their first location in Harlingen, Texas, in 1992. The regimen was simple: a complete thirty-minute workout three days a week and a temporary dieting method that produced permanent results in a supportive environment. The concept was an overwhelming success, and in 1995 the first Curves franchise opened. In just eight years, Curves has grown from one franchise to more than six thousand. Curves is now the world's largest fitness franchise, and the fastest-growing franchise organization of any kind.

Carol Colman is the author or coauthor of numerous best-selling health books.